Ripples in the Flow

by the same author

Returning to the Source
Han Dynasty Medical Classics in Modern Clinical Practice
Z'ev Rosenberg
Edited by Daniel Schrier
Foreword by Sabine Wilms
ISBN 978 1 84819 348 2
eISBN 978 0 85701 306 4

of related interest

Extraordinary Chinese Medicine
The Extraordinary Vessels, Extraordinary Organs, and the Art of Being Human
Thomas Richardson with William Morris
ISBN 978 1 84819 419 9
eISBN 978 0 85701 371 2

A Comprehensive Guide to Daoist Nei Gong
Damo Mitchell
Foreword by Paul Mitchell
ISBN 978 1 84819 410 6
eISBN 978 0 85701 372 9

Heart Shock
Diagnosis and Treatment of Trauma with Shen-
Hammer and Classical Chinese Medicine
Ross Rosen
Foreword by Dr. Leon Hammer
ISBN 978 1 84819 373 4
eISBN 978 0 85701 330 9

Treating Emotional Trauma with Chinese Medicine
Integrated Diagnostic and Treatment Strategies
CT Holman, M.S., L.Ac.
ISBN 978 1 84819 318 5
eISBN 978 0 85701 271 5

The Art and Practice of Diagnosis in Chinese Medicine
Nigel Ching
ISBN 978 1 84819 314 7
eISBN 978 0 85701 267 8

RIPPLES IN THE FLOW

Reflections on Vessel Dynamics in the Nàn Jīng 難經

Z'EV ROSENBERG

Edited by DANIEL SCHRIER
Foreword by LONNY S. JARRETT, M.Ac.

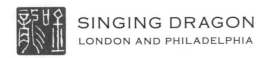

SINGING DRAGON
LONDON AND PHILADELPHIA

First published in 2020
by Singing Dragon
an imprint of Jessica Kingsley Publishers
73 Collier Street
London N1 9BE, UK
and
400 Market Street, Suite 400
Philadelphia, PA 19106, USA

www.singingdragon.com

Library of Congress Cataloging in Publication Data
A CIP catalog record for this book is available from the Library of Congress

British Library Cataloguing in Publication Data
A CIP catalogue record for this book is available from the British Library

ISBN 978 0 85701 391 0
eISBN 978 0 85701 396 5

Printed and bound in the United States

SUSTAINABLE FORESTRY INITIATIVE

Certified Chain of Custody
Promoting Sustainable Forestry
www.sfiprogram.org
SFI-01268

SFI label applies to the text stock

Underground Rivers of Ambient Rhythm

Meditations on the *Nán Jīng* 難經

Under my fingertips
Rivers ebb and flow
Bubbling springs emerge
Winds rise and fall, shift direction

Emotions of conflict are revealed.
Internal viscera respond,
With rhythms that expand and contract,
Revealing their secrets to the mindful physician.

The internal landscape,
With its rhythms, beats, harmonies and
Chaotic manifestations,
Reveals degrees of health and disconnection.

Once revealed,
The needles and herbs awaken resonance,
and body/mind intelligence, restoring
the *zhēn qì* 真氣/true qì.

In the *Nán Jīng* 難經,
These underground rivers form
"A ring without end," a symphonic orchestration
Of mind, heart, emotion, flesh, sinew, viscera and bone.

All this under my fingertips. The life
flowing through my patients,
Revealed to my hands.

Z'ev Rosenberg,
Node of xiǎo hán 小寒/small cold, San Diego, 2019

Contents

Foreword

Don't listen with your ears, listen with your mind. No, don't listen with your mind, but listen with your spirit. Listening stops with the ears, the mind stops with recognition, but spirit is empty and waits on all things. The way gathers in emptiness alone. Emptiness is the fasting of the mind.

Zhuāng Zǐ 莊子[1]

Above all else, pulse diagnosis is a form of listening. "Shutting the doors and windows," letting go of all that might obscure connection between fingertip, heart, and mind through the cultivated touch of pulse diagnosis, we gain access to the patient's subtle depths. Through such listening, we hear the murmurings of processes whose unaltered flow may lead to the misfortune of future suffering. Hence, it is significantly through pulse diagnosis that Chinese medicine attains its status as the world's premiere preventive medicine. When disease is already manifest, the pulse imparts to us a nuanced picture of history, current manifestation, and potential future outcomes.

In Z'ev Rosenberg's second book, *Ripples in the Flow: Reflections on Vessel Dynamics in the Nàn Jīng*, he takes us on a journey through pulse diagnosis as discussed in the Classics. Z'ev is a master scholar-physician, and his insights are compelling as he flushes out the vertical and lateral dimensions of the

---

1   Zhuangzi and Watson 1964: 54

pulse, elaborating its qualities in the context of time, location, and season. In his pursuit of expounding the ecological nature of Chinese medicine, Z'ev impresses on us the principle that humanity and nature are one. He emphasizes the importance of understanding time and place as the context for the expression of all phenomena. Facial colors, pulse qualities, and other diagnostic findings all have their appropriate presentation. It is when such findings are displaced that "evil," commensurate with illness, is indicated.

We can use *Ripples in the Flow* as a companion reader to Paul Unschuld's authoritative translations of many of the texts cited here. Reading side by side, we can go directly to the source material, contemplating the translation and relevant commentaries. In this, Z'ev has generously provided us with a wonderfully condensed and accessible window, not just into the world of classical pulse diagnosis, but also into the method of how a seasoned scholar organizes such material into a coherent picture of meaning and application.

A master practitioner himself, Z'ev concludes by elaborating his use of the principles in the text with six intriguing case studies.

Application of pulse is an essential skill sadly neglected today by our teaching institutions and practitioners alike. *Ripples in the Flow* is an important contribution to a growing literature seeking to rectify this oversight.

Nèi Jīng 內經 commentator Wáng Bīng 王冰 asserts that, "To be able to transmit essence and spirit, only the sages who have attained the Way are able to do this."[2] In *Ripples in the Flow*, Z'ev Rosenberg continues to transmit to us the essence and spirit of his devotion to the path of medicine.

Lonny S. Jarrett, M.Ac.
Author of Nourishing Destiny, The Inner Tradition of Chinese
Medicine and The Clinical Practice of Chinese Medicine

---

2   Unschuld and Tessenow 2011: 61

Acknowledgements

There are several individuals I'd like to thank for contributing, directly or indirectly, to this latest work. My initial interest in the *Nán Jīng* 難經 was spurred back in the 1970s in Boulder, Colorado, by meeting Michael Broffman, L.Ac., of the Pine St. Clinic in San Anselmo, California, whose teacher in Taiwan based his practice of Chinese medicine on the *Nán Jīng* 難經. When I moved to Boulder in 1983, I befriended Donn Hayes, L.Ac., who studied Chinese medicine in Okinawa with a teacher who also relied on the *Nán Jīng* 難經. In 1987, Paul Unschuld published one of the earliest full translations of a Chinese medical classic, the *Nan Ching: The Classic of Difficulties*, and I read and reread this text at least 25 times over the next 30 years, until he updated it in 2016. This little book on *Nán Jīng* 難經 vessel dynamics is designed, with Paul's approval, as a companion work to his translation, providing new insights and applications of the material there. Daniel and I are eternally grateful for his support.

I'd like to thank my wife, Edith, for always being there during (what is for me) the difficult task of writing down these words—spreading dictionaries, texts, paper, iPads and Mac books across the dinner table as I attempted to write this book. And special thanks and gratitude to Daniel Schrier, DOM, L.Ac., my trusty colleague and editor, who has made it possible for me to get out two books in less than a year. Look out for further works that are in the pipeline! I also want to thank Anne Shelton Crute L.Ac., DAOM, for providing essential practitioner feedback, which allowed me to expand the text with relevant material on the clinical utility of vessel dynamics, along with my daughter-in-law Annie Perkins-Rosenberg for the awesome cover art and vessel diagram.

INTRODUCTION

吾生也有涯，而知也无涯。以有涯隨无涯，殆已；已而為
知者，殆而已矣

There is a limit to our life, but to knowledge there is no limit.
With what is limited to pursue after what is unlimited is a
perilous thing; and when, knowing this, we still seek the increase
of our knowledge, the peril cannot be averted.

Zhuāng Zǐ 莊子 Inner Chapters 3
What Matters is the Nourishing of Life[1]

Ripples in the Flow: Reflections on Vessel Dynamics in the Nàn Jīng
難經 is not a pulse manual or a method text, but a compendium
and commentary that allows the practitioner to develop their
own method from the information provided. This text is the
result of my personal study, teaching, and clinical application
of the core chapters on vessel diagnosis in the *Nán Jīng* 難經,
refined over a 30-year period. The *Nán Jīng* 難經 is, according
to Paul Unschuld, "the classic of systematic correspondence"
as applied to diagnosis and treatment. The first 23 difficulties
of the *Nán Jīng* 難經 are a virtual manual of vessel diagnosis,
examining all of the parameters of depth, length, qualities, five
phase relationships, viscera/bowel, channel/network vessel
and season. *Ripples in the Flow: Reflections on Vessel Dynamics
in the Nán Jīng* is designed as a commentary on these essential

---

1   Legge n.d.: https://ctext.org/zhuangzi/nourishing-the-lord-of-life

vessel chapters, as a teaching text, and as a clinical manual for practitioners of acupuncture, moxibustion, and herbal medicine. It will be especially useful for practitioners of five phase approaches to Chinese and Asian medical systems, as it will provide clear classical references for the knowledge that they have been taught in their formal training.

The *Nán Jīng* 難經 largely teaches about the role of time in medicine, in reshaping our clinical gaze by training our minds to view reality from a different perspective. It also reflects on life during the Han dynasty, when humanity measured time not digitally, but from observing the stars and planets, and transformations in the appearance of plants and animals, seasons, the ocean tides, and qualities of light and sound.

Examination of the vessels (*mài zhěn* 脈診) is one of the foundations of the *Nán Jīng* 難經, and formalized the "inch mouth" *cùn kǒu* 寸口 position as a systematic approach to doing so. Vessel diagnosis is our main instrument for measuring transformations of time by tracking flows, changes, movements, rhythms, and qualities as described in the maps developed by the Han dynasty medical sages. The *Nán Jīng* 難經 contains a series of maps that measure the timing of human life in resonance with nature.

The *Nán Jīng* 難經, like other Chinese philosophical and medical classics, is meant to be studied over time, and contemplated to apprehend its simple but profound meaning. It is a guidebook meant to inspire the physician by providing a compass by which to measure one's clinic strategies and results. It is a fulcrum around which the day-to-day practice of Chinese medicine can be hinged. The text is not only a guide to medical practice, it is a meditation on life and nature. We learn that the practice of medicine is as much a way of life as a profession. The *Nán Jīng* 難經 teaches us pattern-based thinking, invoking multiple perspectives on human life in the natural world and cosmos. These patterns may create health or illness, and underneath all the changes in life is the thread of *yīn yáng* and the five phases (*wǔ xíng* 五行). Studying the *Nán Jīng* 難經 will help us build a strong foundation for the practice of Chinese medicine in the 21st century.

The *Nán Jīng* 難經, is a source for vessel dynamics, from which I have drawn much of the information for this text. I have also drawn on material from other seminal Han dynasty medical classics, such as the *Mài Jīng* 脈經/Pulse Classic, the *Shāng Hán Lùn* 傷寒論 pulse chapters, *Sù Wèn* 素問, and *Líng Shū* 靈樞, which are closely related to the material in the *Nán Jīng* 難經. This text is organized as my commentary on the essential pulse chapters in the Nán Jīng 難經, using the Paul Unschuld translation and original Chinese text. This text can be used as a companion to his work.

Z'ev Rosenberg, L.Ac.
San Diego, California, December, 2018

CHAPTER 1

BACKGROUND TO NÁN JĪNG 難經 VESSEL DIAGNOSIS

Only the musically trained could truly know the pulse, because the pulse is of a musical nature.

Ibn Sina on the pulse[1]

Before we delve into specific chapters of the *Nán Jīng* 難經, a historical background to vessel dynamics will be useful. In all pre-modern, literate medical traditions, reading movement in the vessels was and remains the primary diagnostic tool used to read the health, constitution, and illnesses of patients. Each tradition has developed a system of pulse diagnosis as an expression of a comprehensive systematic approach to medicine, with the body/mind seen as a microcosm of heavenly and earthly forces. While it is clinically necessary and useful to focus on a systematic approach, a broad historical background to how the pulse was utilized in the other great medical traditions (Greco/Arabic medicine based on the four humors, Ayurvedic medicine, and Tibetan medicine), as well as unique expressions based on the Chinese medical tradition in Japan, Korea, and other Asian countries, is very useful to gain a broader, more contextual understanding. One will quickly come to the conclusion that reading the pulse (movement in the vessels) was absolutely essential as one of the main diagnostic tools in all literate

---

1   Kuriyama 2011: 81

medical cultures. Paul Unschuld translates *mài* 脈 in this context as "movement in the vessels." His reason for doing so is to avoid the Western mind's tendency to focus on structures (such as arteries and veins) and to focus on flows and transformations.

Mài zhěn 脈診/vessel examination is an art as well as a science, requiring skills of ascertaining dynamics, flow, rhythm, frequency and tone. As we will see in *Nán Jīng* 難經 1, where the primacy of the *cùn kǒu* 寸口/inch mouth position for vessel diagnosis is established, there is a close relationship between movements in the vessel and breathing rhythms. In a closely allied medical tradition, Dr. Vasant Lad, the Ayurvedic pulse master, teaches his students to practice pranayama each morning before reading patients' pulses.

It is useful to look at *Sù Wèn* 素問 17, which is the original source text that explains how the pulses systems in the *Nèi Jīng* 內經 were developed. These multiple systems included: 1) *cùn kǒu* 寸口/*rén yíng* 人迎 outlined in *Líng Shū* 靈樞 chapter 9, which is based on reading and comparing pulse strength, quality, and rhythm between the neck/*rén yíng mài* 人迎脈/*rén yíng* 人迎 pulse and the *cùn kǒu* 寸口/wrist pulse; 2) pulses in three sections of the body, upper middle and lower, hands and feet; and 3) *cùn kǒu* 寸口 pulse, fully developed in the *Nán Jīng* 難經. It is this third system of vessel diagnosis which we will focus on in this pulse manual.

In cultures that lived according to astronomical, seasonal, and agricultural rhythms, the physicians often lived in small villages and saw their patients for pulse readings in the early morning. This was the optimum time for doing so, as this is the time when *yīn* and *yáng* were balanced. In modern times, where daily life rhythms are often distorted by work/sleep schedule disruptions, digital time clocks, and travel, we will need to calculate the departure from this standard accordingly, in order to have accurate pulse readings.

Vessel movement descriptions rely on a qualitative observation of nature and its cycles, rather than quantitative measurements.

As with the time of dawn, when *yīn* and *yáng* are optimally balanced, pre-industrial human beings lived intimately with nature and viewed the world through phenomena such as winds, flowing streams, leafing trees, changes in animal behavior, and movements of birds. We see this with Lǐ Shí-zhēn's 李時珍 explanation of how a floating pulse (*fú mài* 浮脈) should feel, like "a subtle breeze blowing across the down of a bird's back. It is quiet and whispering, like falling elm pods, like wood floating in water, like scallion leaves rolled lightly between the fingers."[2]

---

2   Bray, Dorofeeva-Lichtmann, and Métailié 2007: 61

CHAPTER 2

DECODING THE NÁN JĪNG 難經
Clinical Gaze, Diagnosis, and Practicum

An important factor in understanding Han dynasty medical texts, specifically the *Nán Jīng* 難經, is what medical anthropologist Michel Foucault called the "clinical gaze."[1] Before any treatment, diagnosis, or treatment, it is imperative that a physician views the patient through their own eyes, interpreting what is seen through *li lùn* 理論/theory/principle. The Han dynasty Chinese were fond of interpreting the universe through prime numbers. In the *Nán Jīng* 難經, the number five as expressed through progressive *biàn huà* 變化/transformations through five stages is the predominant numerical basis for understanding human life, health, disease, and the relationship of humanity to nature and the universe. *Wǔ xíng* 五行/five phase principle runs as a common thread throughout the *Nán Jīng* 難經, as an organizing principle for all diagnostic and clinical data. The *Nán Jīng* 難經 system of acupuncture treatment is based on the *wǔ shū xué* 五輸穴/five transporting holes, each associated with a particular phase or *yuán xué* 原穴/source hole, as described in *Nán Jīng* 難經 68.[2]

---

1   For more information refer to Michel Foucault's *The Birth of the Clinic: An Archaeology of Medical Perception* (1973) https://news.northwestern. edu/stories/2013/06/opinion-health-blog-kandula-. "In The Birth of the Clinic, Foucault describes the 'clinical gaze,' which is when the physician perceives the patient as a body experiencing symptoms, instead of as a person experiencing illness."

2   Unschuld (*Nán Jīng*) 2016: 487

The movement in the vessels, palpation of the abdomen, which are described in *Nán Jīng* 難經 16, and visual phenomena (sense organs, skin, complexion, color) are all based on five phase theory (*wǔ xing xue shuō* 行學說).

The Chinese philosopher-scientists observed that nature revealed these numerical patterns. For example, we observe that bees create hexagonal hives. They have developed uniquely patterned eyes and secretions which allow them to sense their environment, specifically blossoms, in order to be able to pollinate and produce honey. These numerical patterns in nature were tapped to understand the relationship of human beings to this wondrous natural world. Physicians developed a multi-dimensional, spatial orientation to channels, such as the *qí jīng bā mài* 奇經八脈/eight extraordinary vessels, discussed in *Nán Jīng* 難經 28, which form an octahedral structure that includes the 12 regular channels, and shares *xué* 穴/holes with those channels, as seen in Figure 2.1.

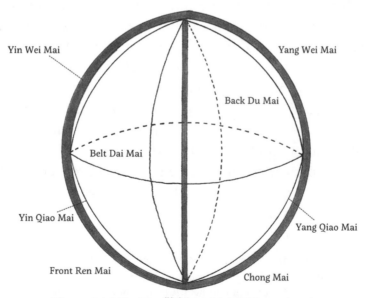

Figure 2.1: Nán Jīng 難經 28 *Multi-Dimensional and Spatial Orientation to Channels*

The relationship of acupuncture holes in the *Nán Jīng* 難經 is described by Dr. Yoshio Manaka as "isophasal," meaning that "certain acupoints on the surface of the body have some similar property, of something functional in common with all other points on the body surface that belong to that phase."[3] Isophasality in turn ties in all of the diagnostic information gained through sound, smell, touch (palpation), vision (*sè* 色/color), and questioning. Accordingly, the physician chooses the proper hole according to *bǔ* 補/supplementation and *xiè* 瀉/drainage, season, use of *yuán xué* 原穴/source holes, *sān jiāo* 三膲/triple burner location (upper, middle, and lower, *Nán Jīng* 難經 31), and *wǔ yùn liù qì* 五運六氣/five movements and six *qì* (circadian cycles). It is clear, when studying the *Nán Jīng* 難經, that this is primarily an internal medicine text, designed to treat *xié qì* 邪氣/evil qì from either *wài gǎn* 外感/external contractions or disruptions of the internal five phase cycles of visceral systems (*nèi shāng* 內傷/internal injury/damage). Only if one does not study the Han dynasty medical classics will one restrict in one's mind the discipline of acupuncture and moxibustion to the treatment of musculoskeletal disorders (affecting what the *Líng Shū* 靈樞 described as *jīn jīng* 筋經/sinew channels).

Nán Jīng 難經 77 stresses the strategy of preventing illness through treatment with acupuncture by reading the vessels and finding the specific imbalances of the five viscera, six bowels, twelve regular and eight extraordinary channels. "The superior practitioner initiates a cure where there is no disease yet; yet the mediocre practitioner treats where there is a disease already."[4] The emphasis is on preventing disease from arising by eliminating underlying disharmonies of *yīn* and *yáng*, and *wǔ xíng* 五行/five phases.

In *Nán Jīng* 難經 69 and 75, these strategies are described in detail, such as "in the case of depletion, supplement the respective

---

3   Manaka, Itaya and Birch 1995: 89
4   Unschuld (*Nán Jīng*) 2016: 532

channel's mother. In the case of repletion, drain the respective channel's child."[5] *Nán Jīng* 難經 75 states "in the case of repletion in the eastern regions and depletion in the western regions, drain the southern regions and supplement the northern regions,"[6] a most sophisticated strategy utilizing the *shēng* 生/generation and *kè* 克/destruction cycles (see Figure 2.2).

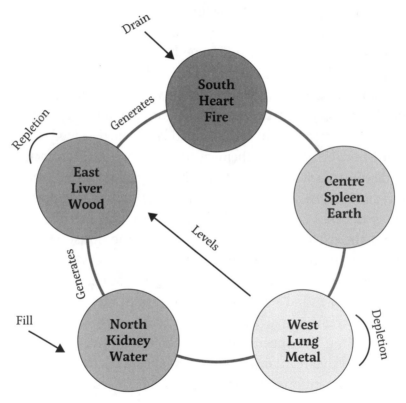

Figure 2.2: Nàn Jīng 難經 *75 Explanation of Shēng* 生/
Generation and kè 克/Destruction Cycle[7]

---

5   ibid: 492

6   ibid: 536

7   Adapted from chart on page 522 in Paul Unschuld's : *Nàn Jīng: The Classic of Difficult Issues*

The channel system as understood in the *Nán Jīng* 難經, via the *wǔ shū xué* 五輸穴/five transporting holes, is based on potentialities of *qì* and blood at different distal and proximal locations on the channels. First of all, depending on the nature of the channel, one needs to determine the relative contents in terms of blood and *qì*, as outlined in *Líng Shū* 靈樞 78, *On the Nine Needles*. Second, each of the five transporting points has a relationship with hand and foot channels, in terms of a relationship of *qì*. The distance from the central trunk on the limbs determines the potentiality of the *xué* 穴/acupuncture hole, so in other words, *hé xué* 合穴/ sea points at the articulations of knees and elbows resonate with each other, just as *jǐng xué* 井穴/well points resonate with each other at the tips of toes and fingers. The channels, which carry *qì* 氣 and *xuè* 血, may be replete or vacuous. This can be felt through palpating *cùn kǒu* 寸口 vessel dynamics. A replete vessel movement will be long and extend past the normal *cùn guān chǐ* 寸關尺 positions, and indicates that the channels are "lengthened." A vacuous vessel movement will be short and fail to fill the associated position(s), meaning that the channels are "shortened." One can see this by viewing the sense organs, as described in *Líng Shū* 靈樞 47; a patient with large, intense, "popping" eyes will often have a replete liver and *jué yīn* 厥陰 channel; a patient with sunken, small, and dim eyes will often have a liver *qì* or *xuè* 血/blood depletion and shortened, thin vessel movements indicating a depleted *jué yīn* 厥陰 channel.

The physician can adjust the flow, intensity, and resonance of the channels using the *wǔ shū xué* 五輸穴/five transporting holes, and read the condition of the channel system relying on the vessel dynamics system described in *Nán Jīng* 難經 15, 16, and 18.

CHAPTER 3

NÁN JĪNG 難經 1–3

Vessel Architecture and Relationship to Time

故五十度復會於手太陰。寸口者，五藏六府之所終始，
故法取於寸口也

*Because the contents of the vessels meet again, after 50 passages,
with the inch opening, this section is the beginning and the end
of the movement of the contents of the vessels through the body's
five yin viscera and six bowels. Hence, the patterns are obtained
from the inch opening.[1]*

I. The first three chapters of the *Nán Jīng* 難經 emphasize
the importance of location and position over physiology. It is
not the actual vessel that is palpated that is of importance, or
its contents, but the movement and flow of substances along
and within these *jīng mài* 經脈/vessels that is significant: "The
meaning of what the fingers felt, depended on where they [are]
felt."[2] In other words, in contrast to vessel diagnosis as described
by Galen in Greco-Arabic medicine, Chinese vessel diagnosis is
qualitative, rather than quantitative. It has everything to do with
timing, position in the *cùn kǒu* 寸口 relative to different parts
of the body, but also reflects the *wǔ zhì* 五志/five sentiments
(emotions) that are connected with the *wǔ zàng* 五臟/five

---

1   Unschuld (*Nán Jīng*) 2016: 58
2   Kuriyama 2011: 40

yīn viscera. Lǐ Dōng-yuán 李東垣 stated that "Although the three fingers are separated by mere hairbreadths, the diseases they indicate are a thousand leagues apart."[3] The vessel positions are like the Japanese landscape paintings done on a single grain of rice. An incredible amount of detail is condensed in a tiny area, and by gently rotating the fingers, one can find out a great deal of clinical information.

Here we will learn how to understand and calculate the circulation of *wèi qì* 衛氣 and *yíng qì* 營氣 in resonance with the breath. In this way, the practitioner can palpate the vessels to read the condition of the body/mind at any time of day. In the *Líng Shū* 靈樞, the day is divided into four segments: "The morning is spring. Noon is summer. Sunset is autumn. Midnight is winter."[4] As the *yíng* 營 and *wèi* 衛 circulate through the *yáng/*exterior and *yīn/*interior aspects of the body, the qualities of the movements in the vessels change. According to the *Sù Wèn* 素問, the vessel movement is most balanced just before dawn (or as described in Tibetan medicine, "as the sun's first rays appear, but do not strike the plains, just the hills."[5] In *Sù Wèn* 素問 17, it states:

> As a rule it is at dawn, before the *yīn qì* has begun its movement, before the *yáng qi* is dispersed, before beverages and food have been consumed, before the conduit vessels are filled to abundance, when the *luò mài* 絡脈/network vessels are balanced, before *qì* and the blood move in disorder, that, hence, one can diagnose an abnormal movement in the vessels."[6]

On this, Lǐ Zhōng-zǐ 李中梓 comments:

> The *wèi* 衛 and *yíng qì* 營氣 of the human body, during daytime they pass through the *yáng* section, during nighttime they

---

3   ibid: 40
4   Unschuld (*Líng Shū*) 2016: 426
5   Dhonden and Hopkins 1986: 76–77
6   Unschuld and Tessenow 2011: 273–274

pass through the *yīn* section. In early morning they convene at the *cùn kǒu* 寸口/inch opening. Hence the examination of the movement in the vessels should be carried out in the early morning, when the *yīn qì* 陰氣 is tranquil and does not yet move, when the *yáng qì* 陽氣 is about to abound and has yet dispersed, and before food and beverages have been taken.[7]

In *Sù Wèn* 素問 23, we see the following descriptions of movement in the vessels, which is also described in *Nán Jīng* 難經 18.

> The phenomena reflecting the five [movements in the] vessels: The liver [movement in the] vessels is string[-like]. The heart [movement in the] vessels is hook[-like]. The spleen [movement in the] vessels is intermittent. The lung [movement in the] vessels is hair[-like]. The kidney [movement in the] vessels is stone[-like]."[8]

According to Wáng Bīng 王冰, the meaning of *dài* 代/intermittent is not limited to a vessel dynamic that stops and starts, but also "alternating between big and small," or "substituting itself in the course of the four seasons."[9] This can mean: 1) interruption in the regular rhythm of vessel movement (the usually accepted definition) 2) changes in the manifestation of qualities while palpating the vessels, or 3) changes in vessel dynamics synchronous with seasonal *qì*. In other words, a vessel movement in summer time intermittently manifests a wiry or spring-like quality.

Einstein taught that "our idea of time is something we abstract from our experience with rhythmic phenomena: heartbeats, planetary rotations and revolutions, the ticking of clocks".[10] And our relationship with time in the modern world is very different from that in the Han dynasty, when the

---

7   Unschuld and Tessenow 2011: 273–274
8   ibid: 410
9   ibid: 410
10   Holt 2018

Nán Jīng 難經 was written. The Han Chinese were philosophers and scientists, and dealt with a world perceived through their own minds and senses, in a natural world not yet influenced by industrial technology or digital devices. The measuring device for movement of *qì* 氣 in the body/mind was the clepsydra or water clock, synchronous with inhalation and exhalation. With each inhalation, the *qì* 氣 moved three *cùn* 寸; with each exhalation, the *qì* 氣 moved three *cùn* 寸. The *Nán Jīng* 難經 states that there are 13,500 breaths in a 24-hour period, and that the *wèi qì* 衛氣 and the *yíng qì* 營氣 precede through 50 passages, 25 during the *yáng* period (daytime), and 25 during the *yīn* period (nighttime). The *qì* primarily circulated from *yáng* at the surface during the daytime, to *yīn* on the interior during the nighttime, tempered by the length of day in the different seasons. The *wèi qì* 衛氣/defense *qì* circulated 50 times per day using these measurements, and circulated to replenish the five *yīn* viscera, ending at the kidneys just before dawn before again moving upwards and outwards towards the exterior. This natural "irrigation system" was again measured against the clepsydra's dripping water down through 200 markings.

The result of the industrial and digital revolutions has been to speed up human life in relationship to the natural world, and specifically to one's own body and mind. Journeys across continents or oceans used to take weeks, now they take hours. One can fly from winter in Chicago to summer in Sydney in less than 24 hours. Our circadian rhythms have been altered and distorted in many ways by high speed travel, information processing, changes in work/scholastic and natural rhythms such as eating, sleeping, sex, and physical exercise.

In my first book, *Returning to the Source: Han Dynasty Medical Classics in Modern Clinical Practice*, I described this modern phenomenon as "degrees of disconnection." The seminal chapters of the *Sù Wèn* 素問 (1–6) illustrate the primal rhythms of season, day, and how to live in harmony with environmental changes that occur regularly through days, months, seasons, years, lunar and solar cycles. The *Nán Jīng* 難經 records for us the vessel dynamics that reflect normal seasonal changes, and then we can measure digressions from those normative states in terms of our lifestyles. The *Sù Wèn* 素問 teaches us optimum activities for each season, in terms of work, sleep, clothing, food, activity, and state of consciousness (reflective or active). Digressions from these seasonal rhythms lead to illnesses in the following seasons. In *Sù Wèn* 素問 3, it says "if one was harmed in winter by cold, in spring he will develop a warmth disease."[11] This *shāng hán* 傷寒/cold damage was caused by not living according to the requirements of the winter season (proper clothing, sleep schedule, diet, activity, and behavior).

In order to learn and practice *mài zhěn* 脈診/vessel examination, the physician must be aware of these embedded cycles in nature, and observe how the patient diverges or conforms to these cycles. In turn, this will manifest in aberrations in the vessel movements, rhythms and qualities. The physician him/herself has to embrace the lifestyle described in the *Sù Wèn* 素問 in order to be aware of these "degrees of disconnection" that manifest in the vessel movements. And, in the clinic, the physician needs to create an environment where they can disconnect from the limitations of digital time and return to the rhythms of breath, solar and lunar cycles. The more detached one is from nature, the more disconnection from *zhèng qì* 正氣/correct qì and ideal health. It says in *Sù Wèn* 素問 13:

> When the people of later generations treated a disease, the treatments were not based in the four seasons. They no longer knew the significance of sun and moon. They did not recognize whether the *qì* moved contrary to or followed its proper course.[12]

---

11 Unschuld and Tessenow 2011: 79
12 Unschuld and Tessenow 2011: 227

We see that even historically it was difficult to remain in this awareness. Today, practitioners of Chinese medicine rarely are aware of this!

Later it says in *Sù Wèn* 素問 13 to "Close the door and shut the windows, tie yourself to the patient."[13] This means creating an environment where the patient feels safe, peaceful, and able to participate in the treatment and healing process. It also admonishes the physician to be focused on the needs of the patient to the exclusion of outside sounds and distractions, and internal wanderings of their thoughts.

The movement of *qì* through the five phases, and their associated transport holes, channels and visceral systems, is said in the *Nán Jīng* 難經 to be like "a ring without end."[14] Because of this, the *cùn kǒu* 寸口/inch opening, position on the wrist is located at Lung 9 (*tài yuān* 太淵/Supreme Abyss), the meeting point of the vessels. This location reflects the movement of *yīn* 陰 and *yáng* 陽, *yíng* 營 and *wèi* 衛, through circadian cycles associated with lunar, solar, 24-hour, and seasonal cycles.

With the *cùn kǒu* 寸口/inch opening now established as *the* location to palpate the vessels, we are now ready to examine the dimensions of reading the vessels with all of their contained depths and nuances; as opposed to on individual vessel sites which classically were nine palpable locations on the body divided into three positions of heaven, human, and earth.

II. *Nàn Jīng* 難經 2 and 3 divide the *cùn kǒu* 寸口 vessel dynamic into three regions: *cùn*寸/inch, *guān* 關/gate/bar, and *chǐ* 尺/foot/cubit, the inch being the realm of *yáng*, the cubit being the realm of *yīn*, and the bar the separation between the two. The dimensionality of the movement in the vessels is established in these two chapters. This method is known as the *sān bù* 三部/three sectors method. As some of the discussion in these chapters seems to indicate, specifically on the length of

---

13 ibid: 230
14 ibid: 170

each sector in *cùn* 寸, originally the length of the arm from wrist crease to elbow crease was used for palpation and diagnosis (see Figure 3.1). At these locations (*cùn* 寸/*guān* 關/*chǐ* 尺), *mài xiàng* 脈象/vessel images were interpreted in relationship to the upper, middle, and lower burners, their contents in terms of *zàng* 臟/ viscera and *fǔ* 腑/bowels, and the locations of channel flows in these regions, including the 12 main channels and *qí jīng bā mài* 奇經八脈/eight extraordinary vessels.

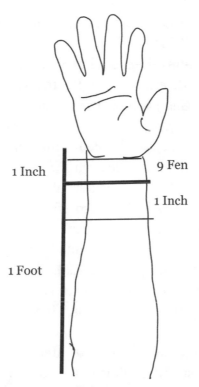

1 Inch

9 Fen

1 Inch

1 Foot

Figure 3.1: Nán Jīng 難經 2 Foot Inch Vessel Section

One approach to vessel diagnosis uses a method that primarily reads the *cùn* 寸 and *chǐ* 尺 positions, and views the *guān* 關 as a dividing line or barrier between the two. According to Huá Shòu 滑壽, a commentator on the *Nàn Jīng* 難經, the *guān* 關/ gate "is the dividing line formed by the elevated bone behind the palms. It acts as a borderline between the two areas of *yin* and *yang*."[15] In *Nàn Jīng* 難經 2, it states "the foot and inch is the section where one examines depth and surface, smoothness and roughness, in order to know where a disease has emerged."[16]

Nàn Jīng 難經 18 has clearly established the tripartite *cùn* 寸/*guān* 關/*chǐ* 尺 positions as the basis of *mài zhěn* 脈診/ vessel examination. So, the purpose of this chapter is simply to magnify what occurs between the upper and lower, *yáng* and *yīn* sectioning of the vessel, rather than the complete picture presented in *Nàn Jīng* 難經 18.

III. In *Nán Jīng* 難經 3, the *guān* 關/gate is seen as a barrier between the *cùn* 寸/inch and *chǐ* 尺/foot positions. The length of these two positions (long or short), and overflowing or not reaching qualities, determine what the text calls *fù* 覆/turnover or *yì* 益/overflow. *Guān* 關/(external) closure and *gé* 格/barrier, according to Katō Bankei,[17] refers to a disease where *yīn*, located in the *chǐ* 尺 realm, and *yáng*, located in the *cùn* 寸 realm, displace each other. This is an example of *nì* 逆/counterflow, where the correct placement of internal/external, upper and lower, and *yīn* and *yáng* qualities is displaced and moves to circumvent the normal order (of *yīn* and *yáng qì*) of the body. When *yīn* is vacuous, *yáng* takes over. When *yáng qì* is vacuous, *yīn* takes over. If *yīn* rises up, *yáng qì* cannot descend as the *yīn qì* provides a barrier, leading to external heat with ceaseless sweating, with internal cold, fullness in the chest and inability to take in food. When the *yīn qì* is vacuous, the *yáng qì* descends to the lower burner, causing internal closure and external barrier, leading to internal heat, constipation, difficult urination with exterior cold with cold extremities (*sì nì* 四逆).

Nán Jīng 難經 37 covers the movement of *qì* of the five *yīn* viscera through their associated sense organs, assuring clear sense of taste (spleen), vision (liver), flavors (heart), and hearing (kidneys). It states that when the five *yīn* viscera are not at ease,

15 Unschuld (*Nán Jīng*) 2016: 65
16 ibid: 67
17 ibid: 77

the nine orifices are not passable. So, as long as there is free flow in the *yīn* and *yáng* channels, "*rén qì* 人氣/human *qì* provides the *zàng* and *fǔ* with internal warmth, and moistens the pores (skin) externally."

What is being described above is *qì huà* 氣化/*qì* transformation, the unobstructed ascension of the *qīng qì* 清氣/clear *qì*, and descent of the *zhuó qì* 濁氣/turbid *qì*. When there is obstruction in the middle burner, corresponding to the *guān* 關, it leads to disturbance of normal *qì* transformation, and the organism is disturbed. In addition, if either *yīn* or *yáng* is vacuous, one will fill the position of the other, leading to disharmony between upper and lower burners, interior and exterior. This is a form of *jué* 厥/inversion, where the proper locations of *yīn* and *yáng*, *qì* and blood, above and below "turn over" (*fù* 覆) and subvert the natural order of the body/mind. The normal metabolic, digestive, circulatory, and functional aspects of the organism are all regulated by *qì* transformation, so resolving this middle burner blockage, separating *yáng* from *yīn*, above from below, and leading to *nì* 逆/counterflow or *fù* 覆/turnover or *yì* 溢/overflow, can all be read on the vessels in terms of repletion above, vacuity below, or vacuity above, repletion below. As it says in *Líng Shū* 靈樞 17 (*mài dù* 脈度), "when the *yīn qì* abounds excessively, then the *yáng qì* are unable to circulate."[18] When this happens, you will find external heat and sweating with internal cold, when *yáng qì* cannot descend and *yīn qì* fills up the interior. There can also be internal heat, urinary stoppage and constipation, with cold hands and feet, when the *yīn qì* are blocked inside and *yáng qì* sinks inwards. "*Rén qì* 人氣/human *qì*" here means the *xiàng huà* 相火/ministerial fire that circulates via the *sān jiāo* 三焦/triple burner throughout the organism. It fills all the spaces in the body, circulating warmth (*wèi qì* 衛氣/defensive *qì*) everywhere, and moistening the spaces in the skin with *yíng qì* 營氣/construction *qì*.

---

18 Unschuld (*Nán Jīng*) 2016: 73

As we discussed in *Returning to the Source: Han Dynasty Medical Classics in Modern Clinical Practice*,[19] *qì huà* 氣化/qì transformation and *xiàng huǒ* 相火/ministerial fire are essential principles for understanding classical Chinese medicine, its diagnosis and clinical applications. The correct location and position of *yīn qì* in the interior and lower burner (water, containing dragon fire), *yáng qì* at the exterior and upper burner (fire, containing heart *yīn*) interact in a manner that maintains life and health when normative *qì* transformation is able to function. When *yīn* and *yáng* are inverted and displaced, this is the beginning of disease.

---

19 Rosenberg 2018

CHAPTER 4

NÁN JĪNG 難經 4–5 VESSEL ARCHITECTURE CONTINUED
Yīn Yáng 陰陽 Patterns and Five Depths Vessel Diagnosis

In *Nán Jīng* 難經 Difficult Issue 4, the rhythms of inhalation and exhalation move from exterior to interior and back, from above to below, from *yáng* to *yīn* to *yáng* again. As in *Nán Jīng* 難經 Difficult Issue 1, the channel *qì* corresponds and moves along with respiration. In that chapter, the *yīn* viscera are nourished according to the 24-hour cycle, with 25 movements of *yíng qì* 營氣/construction and *wèi qì* 衛氣/defense *qì* during daylight hours at the exterior, and 25 movements at the interior during the *yīn*/nighttime. Both the lung and heart are associated with the upper burner above the diaphragm, their vessel movements must be distinguished by qualitative analysis: the heart is distinguished by a strong, *sàn* 散/scattering quality, whereas a *sè* 澀/rough and short vessel movement is associated with the lung viscus. Since both the liver and kidney occupy the depth and lower burner, their vessel movements are distinguished by, in case of the liver, a *láo* 牢/firm and *cháng* 長/long quality, and with the kidney, a *ruò* 弱/soft but replete quality when pressed to the bone and gently lifted. The spleen vessel movement, at the center between upper and lower burners, is not given any specific quality in this chapter.

The second part of Difficult Issue 4 of the *Nán Jīng* 難經 discusses vessel movements associated with *sān yáng* 三陽/ *sān yīn* 三陰, the six channels, again differentiating the exterior (three *yáng* channels) from the interior (three *yīn* channels), each with their specific quality (see Figure 4.1). This differentiation was first described in the *Sù Wèn* 素問 Chapter 6, *Discourse on the Division and Unity of Yīn and Yáng (yīn yáng lí hé lùn piān dì liù* 陰陽離合論篇第六). Here we see the *Nán Jīng* 難經 explaining this in terms of depth of the viscus (liver and kidney being the deepest and lowest viscera), and in congruence with its five phase classification of the vessel diagnosis, including the chapter on the five depths, where lung is at the top, the next depth is heart, center is spleen, below that is liver, bone depth is kidney. This model is different from the more commonly used system of vessel diagnosis based on Lǐ Shí-zhēn's 李時珍 *Bīn Hú Mài Xué* 瀕湖脈學/*Creekside Master's Vessel Studies*. Figure 4.2 outlines the differentiation of these vessel qualities.

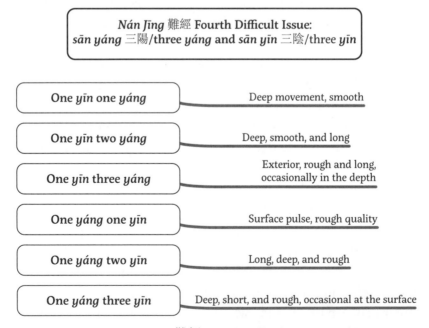

Figure 4.1: Nán Jīng 難經 *Fourth Difficult Issue: sān yáng*
三陽/*three yáng and sān yīn* 三陰/*three yīn*

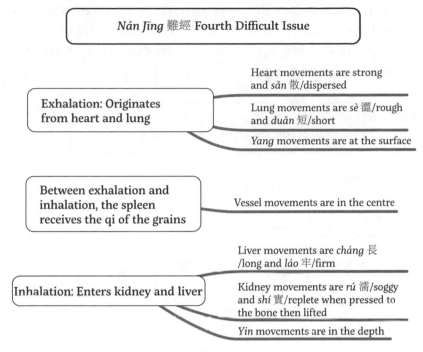

Figure 4.2: Nán Jīng 難經 *Fourth Difficult Issue*

Each of the six vessel movements is differentiated by depth and quality. This allows for further differentiation, established in the first three difficulties by position on the wrist in terms of *cùn* 寸 *guān* 關 *chǐ* 尺/inch, bar and foot/cubit. The *Sù Wèn* 素問 states:

> Hence, in the division and unity of the three yáng [vessels], the major yáng is the opening; the yáng brilliance is the door leaf; the minor yáng is the pivot… Hence, in the division and unity of the three yin, the major yīn is the opening; the ceasing yīn is the door leaf; the minor yīn is the pivot. [1]

An entirely new vessel diagnostic architecture is revealed in *Nán Jīng* 難經 Difficult Issue 5. The vessel is divided longitudinally into five depths, each revealed by "light" to "heavy" pressure, each depth corresponding to a specific viscera. In consecutive

---

1   Unschuld and Tessenow 2011: 131–134

order, from the surface (light pressure, three beans) corresponds to the lungs, to the interior (bone level, kidneys). Following the lungs, the next depth (six beans) corresponds to the heart. This is shown in Figure 4.3.

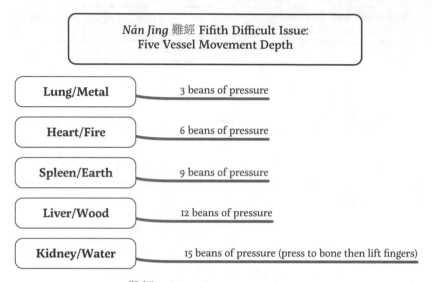

Figure 4.3: Nán Jīng 難經 *Fifth Difficult Issue: Five Vessel Movement Depth*

In *Nán Jīng* 難經 Difficult Issue 4, we saw that the *qì* of lungs and heart, above the diaphragm is associated with exhalation moving towards the exterior, the liver and kidney, below the diaphragm, receives *qì* through inhalation. Between upper and lower burner lies the zone of the spleen, which is activated between the in-breath and out-breath, as befitting its central importance in five phase theory. In five depths vessel diagnosis, the *wǔ zàng* 五臟/ five *yīn* viscera are layered in accordance with this movement of respiration and *qì* from exterior to interior, *yáng* to *yīn* and back to *yáng* again. So, the *Nán Jīng* 難經 is providing yet another map for reading vessel dynamics, one that "stacks" each of the *yīn* viscera by depth and position in the *sān jiāo* 三膲/ triple burner, from above to below. This method, rarely utilized in modern practice except by those physicians trained specifically in *Nán Jīng* 難經 medicine, provides a useful, "architectural" model and map for yet another dimension of diagnostic information that is revealed in the vessel/channel system. In my own practice, I will use this vessel map to determine where specific illnesses are located in terms of specific depths or viscera. It is a complementary model to the *Shāng Hán Lùn's* 傷寒論 *sān yáng* 三陽/ three *yáng*, *sān yīn* 三陰/three *yīn* channel differentiation method.

CHAPTER 5

NÁN JĪNG 難經 6
Yīn Abundance/Yáng Depletion, Yáng Abundance/Yīn Depletion

Difficult Issue 6 discusses the *yīn/yáng* differentiation of vessel dynamics architecture having to do with contrasting vessel qualities between the exterior and the interior, the exterior associated with *yáng*, and the interior associated with *yīn*. The text clearly describes the vessel movements associated with *shí* 實/repletion and *xū* 虛/depletion/vacuity. The purpose here is to authoritatively introduce refinements of vessel dynamics architecture, revealing position, depth, strength, and timing as part of a grid associated with *cùn* 寸, *guān* 關, *chǐ* 尺.

Examining vessel dynamics is often difficult in its study, because of the various schools of thought, methods, and the different qualities and focus of acupuncture/moxibustion and herbal medicine. If we look at these different aspects of vessel dynamics as overlaying maps, we can understand and embrace the different layers of information revealed by using an architectural model. The *Nán Jīng* 難經 lays out for us, step by step, an architectural model that can be accessed from different layers and perspectives. However, the practitioner must first be aware that this information exists, otherwise they will never know it is there.

The approach in the *Nán Jīng* 難經 can be compared with that in other texts focused on vessel dynamics, such as Lǐ Shí-zhēn's 李時珍 *Bīn Hú Mài Xué* 瀕湖脈學, for example, where vessel dynamics reflect humoral and visceral changes in the *sān jiāo* 三膲 and their contents, including the *zàng* 臟/*yīn* viscera, *jīn yè* 津液/fluids, *xuè* 血/blood, and pathological products such as *tán* 痰/phlegm. By contrast, in classics such as the *Zhēn Jiǔ Dà Chéng* 針灸大成/*Systematic Classic of Acupuncture and Moxibustion*, the focus is more on relationships of channels and network vessels to each other, a more "architectural" view. All of these systems are valuable and can be compared to obtaining different maps of a wilderness area before hiking and camping. You can get maps that focus on altitude, rainfall, landmarks, photos of the landscape, or superimpose the maps on each other in more complex maps. It is no different with vessel diagnosis; there are different systems and approaches, but since all of these maps are based on the Han dynasty classics, the maps that are revealed in the *Sù Wèn* 素問, *Líng Shū* 靈樞, *Nán Jīng* 難經, and *Shāng Hán Lùn* 傷寒論 will provide the foundations that are necessary in order to understand later developments.

CHAPTER 6

NÁN JĪNG 難經 7

Arrival of Channel and Seasonal Qì in Vessel Dynamics

> *If he (the physician) has understood this pattern and if (the interrelations of yin and yang, and of the five phases, are clearly in his breast, a physician upon lowering his hands to examine the vessels feels a movement in the vessels corresponding to the season, and he/she immediately knows that is neither a normal movement nor one affected by a disease, but a movement of governing qi through the vessels.*
>
> Zhàng Shì-xián's 悵世賢 commentary on
> Difficult Issue 7 of the *Nán Jīng* 難經[1]

The next step in defining vessel dynamics is revealing the qualities of each of the six channels and their associated time/season in the Chinese calendar. Each of the paired three *yīn* and three *yáng* channels exhibits *wáng qì* 王氣/ruling *qì*/governing *qì*, reflecting the cycle of *shí qì* 時氣/seasonal *qì*, rather than pathology or physiology. These cycles are embedded in vessel dynamics and are read as an underlying "code" in the vessel dynamics. One of our first examinations in vessel dynamics is to read the seasonal *qì* and active channels, which will also reflect in the time of day/24-hour cycle. The *Mài Jīng* 脈經 also establishes the daily cycles of vessel dynamics (see Figure 6.2).

---

1   Unschuld (*Nán Jīng*) 2016: 106

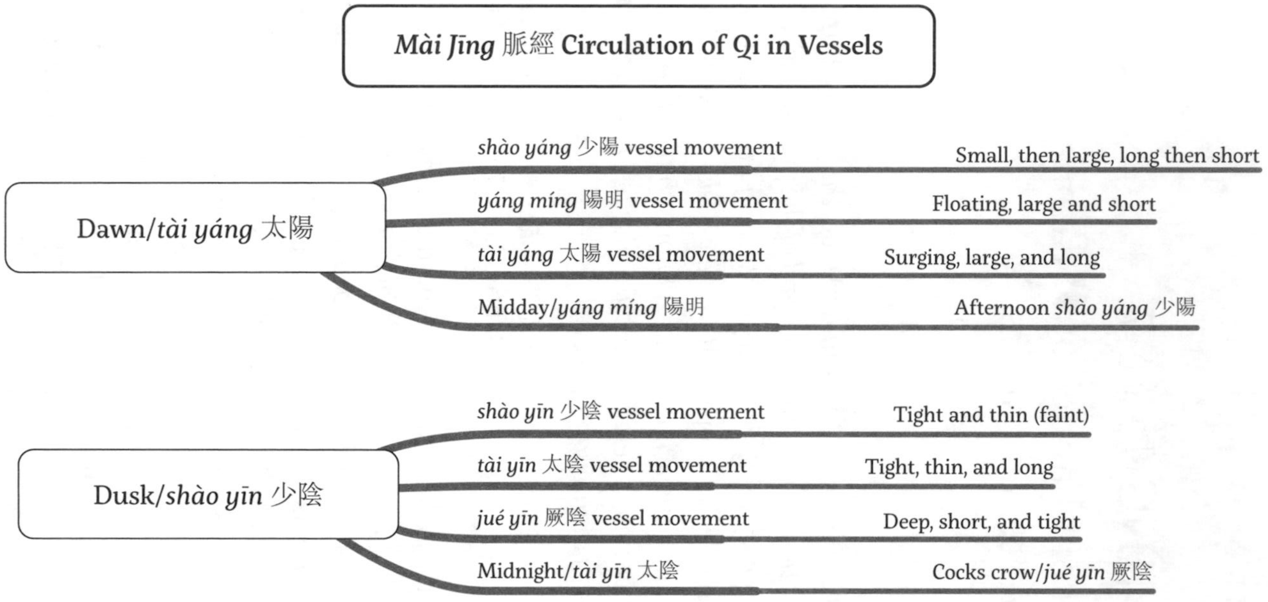

Mài Jīng 脈經 **Circulation of Qi in Vessels**

Dawn/*tài yáng* 太陽

- *shào yáng* 少陽 vessel movement — Small, then large, long then short
- *yáng míng* 陽明 vessel movement — Floating, large and short
- *tài yáng* 太陽 vessel movement — Surging, large, and long
- Midday/*yáng míng* 陽明 — Afternoon *shào yáng* 少陽

Dusk/*shào yīn* 少陰

- *shào yīn* 少陰 vessel movement — Tight and thin (faint)
- *tài yīn* 太陰 vessel movement — Tight, thin, and long
- *jué yīn* 厥陰 vessel movement — Deep, short, and tight
- Midnight/*tài yīn* 太陰 — Cocks crow/*jué yīn* 厥陰

Figure 6.1: Mài Jīng 脈經 Circulation of Qi in Vessels

So we see there are different layers in vessel dynamics to be read that are illustrated in the *Nán Jīng* 難經: 1) *shí qì* 時氣 seasonal *qì;* 2) 24-hour cycles of movement of *yíng* 營 and *wèi* 衛; 3) five phase movements; 4) *wài gǎn* 外感/exterior contractions by environmental changes (wind, cold, damp, summer heat, fire, dryness); 5) *nèi shāng* 內傷/internal damage by emotions, diet, constitutional factors; 6) relationship of *sān jiāo* 三焦/triple burner, upper middle, and lower regions (defined in the *Nán Jīng* 難經 as *shàng* 上/the region above Ren 17 (膻中 *shān zhōng*), *zhōng* 中/the region between Ren 17 and Ren 9 (水分 *shuǐ fēn*) and *xià* 下/the region below the navel; and 7) specific disease entities. Depending on the case, the practitioner looks at what is most prominent at the time and its relation to the above factors. The vessel movement will reveal one or multiple factors that are prominent in the patient's condition. The practitioner doesn't need to look at all of these factors at the same time. He or she can look at what is in the foreground and what is in the background, much like a painting. Often during acumoxa treatments the movement in the vessel will change and factors that were hidden, stresses or emotional upsets, and so on, may allow other factors to come up and be read at that moment. I will often use acupuncture treatment diagnostically, especially back shù points (*bèi shù xué* 背俞穴) to clear up "static" if the vessel seems unclear.

In *Nán Jīng* 難經 Difficult Issue 4, we differentiated the six channel vessels by categorization through qualities of *yīn* and *yáng* (one *yīn*/one *yáng*, one *yīn*/two *yáng*, one *yīn*/three *yáng*, etc.). Now we name each of the three *yīn* and three *yáng* channels with their appropriate dynamic quality and *jiǎ zǐ* 甲子 term, each term a period of two months or 60 days, approximately 360 days for six terms which in turn corresponds to the six paired channels. Each *jiǎ zǐ* 甲子 period has an associated channel, beginning with *shào yáng* 少陽 after the winter solstice. This is followed by *yáng míng* 陽明, *tài yáng* 太陽, *tài yīn* 太陰, *shào yīn* 少陰, and *jué yīn* 厥陰, and back to *shào yáng* 少陽, creating a cyclic movement of *qi* through the seasons in the associated channels (see Figure 6.2).

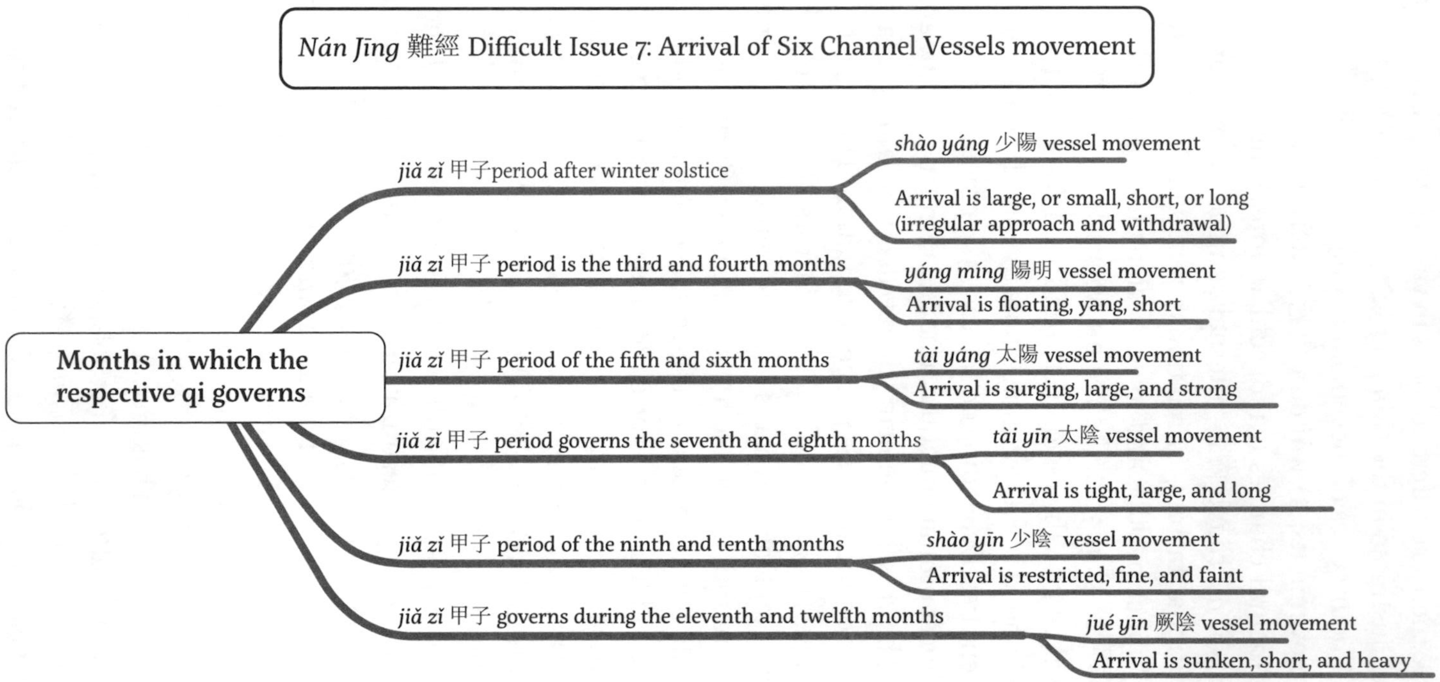

Figure 6.2: *Nán Jīng* 難經 *Difficult Issue 7: Arrival of Six Channel Vessels Movement*

Nán Jīng 難經 Difficult Issue 7: Arrival of Six Channel Vessels movement

Months in which the respective qi governs

jiǎ zǐ 甲子 period after winter solstice

jiǎ zǐ 甲子 period is the third and fourth months

jiǎ zǐ 甲子 period of the fifth and sixth months

jiǎ zǐ 甲子 period governs the seventh and eighth months

jiǎ zǐ 甲子 period of the ninth and tenth months

jiǎ zǐ 甲子 governs during the eleventh and twelfth months

shào yáng 少陽 vessel movement

Arrival is large, or small, short, or long (irregular approach and withdrawal)

yáng míng 陽明 vessel movement

Arrival is floating, yang, short

tài yáng 太陽 vessel movement

Arrival is surging, large, and strong

tài yīn 太陰 vessel movement

Arrival is tight, large, and long

shào yīn 少陰 vessel movement

Arrival is restricted, fine, and faint

jué yīn 厥陰 vessel movement

Arrival is sunken, short, and heavy

Nán Jīng 難經 Difficulty 7 states "the arrival of the *shào yáng* 少陽 is at times *dà* 大/strong/big, at times *shào* 少/minor, at times *cháng* 長/long (extended). According to Lu Guǎng 呂廣, this is due to "*yáng qì* being weak and feeble"[2] (after the winter solstice). As the progression of seasonal *qì* continues, the associated channels are qualitatively associated with the specific *qì* of that time of year. *Yáng míng* 陽明 vessel dynamics are strong, short, and at the surface, as warmth begins to generate and *yáng qì* increases (early spring). *Tài yáng* 太陽 vessel dynamics are vast, strong, and extended, when *yáng qì* is abundant (high summer). In long summer, *tài yīn* 太陰 vessel *qì* dominates, confined, strong, and long/extended. There is still heat and humidity, but the vessel quality is now deeper and more confined as autumn *qì* develops, and yin *qì* predominates. When autumn coolness begins, the *shào yīn* 少陰 vessel dynamics are restricted, having a fine and feeble quality. The *jué yīn* 厥陰 vessel dynamics are the completion of the yearly cycle, as winter condenses water *qì*. *Jué yīn* 厥陰 channel dynamics are described as deep, short, and sinking.

Of course, despite calendrical markings and calculations, seasonal *qì* varies because of *zhǔ qì* 主氣/host and *kè qì* 客氣/guest *qì*, different regions, altitudes, and climates, so we must adjust these calculations to actual observed conditions.

---

2   Unschuld (*Nán Jīng*) 2016: 101

CHAPTER 7

NÀN JĪNG 難經 8 AND 24

Mìng Mén 命門 Dynamics and Severance of the Vessels

I. "All the twelve channels are linked with the *yuán* 原/origin of the *shēng qì* 生氣/vital *qì*."[1] This origin is the *mìng mén* 命門, also called "the moving *qì*" between the kidneys. The *sān jiāo* 三焦/triple burner emerges from this location as well, and the *mìng mén* 命門 constitutes a person's root and foundation. *Nàn Jīng* 難經 8 asks why a patient with normal, balanced vessel dynamics dies, despite having a seemingly healthy vessel movement and circulation. To explain the reasoning behind this, one can compare the patient's *qì* to a vase of cut flowers, which will survive for a short period subsisting on the water in the vase. Its branches and flowers have been cut off from the roots, so that true vital nourishment ceases. This "severance" of the vessels can be applied to human life in terms of original constitution. A person with a weak constitution has weak *jīng* 精/essence and *yuán qì* 原氣/source *qì* to carry out the *yáng* transformations required to maintain life. The *qí jīng bā mài* 奇經八脈/eight extraordinary vessels in particular create the structure on which life forces of heaven and earth embody the human form. At a certain point, the source *qì* and essence "run out of steam," transformation fails, and even though the vessel movements

---

1   Unschuld (*Nàn Jīng*) 2016: 107

appear to be normal, at a certain point they will fail to appear, and life will cease to exist.

Different source texts identify the *mìng mén* 命門 in a slightly different manner. Wú Kūn 吳昆, one of the commentators on the *Sù Wèn* 素問, remarks on *Sù Wèn* 素問 52 that "the gate of life/*mìng mén* 命門 is the *xiàng huǒ* 相火/ministerial fire. The ministerial fire carries out tasks on behalf of the heart ruler. Therefore it is called *xiǎo xīn* 小心/small heart."[2] *Mìng mén* 命門 is the master of the 12 channels, and the *mìng mén huǒ* 命門火 life gate fire contains the igniting spark that awakens *qì huà* 氣化/qì transformation in the 12 channels. Without this (ministerial) fire inside, we cannot exist; it is like a gas stove's pilot light, without which the oven and burners cannot turn on. The ministerial fire warms the body and performs all *huà* 化/transformations, and must not be allowed to go out. It is a type of prenatal fire, immaterial and dwelling in water, a *yáng* manifestation that is embedded between two *yīn* (lines). All of the visceral networks rely on the *mìng mén* 命門 for warmth and nourishment. We use intensive moxibustion, or strong *yáng/shào yīn* 少陰 formulas such as *sì nì tāng*/Frigid Extremities Decoction, *jīn guì shèn qì wán*/Golden Cabinet Kidney Qi Pill or *zhēn wǔ tāng*/True Warrior Decoction to nurture and warm the *yáng qì* and *xiàng huǒ* 相火/ministerial fire with *fù zǐ/Aconiti radix Lateralis, ròu guì/Cinnamomi cortex* and *gān jiāng/Zingiberis rhizoma*.

This, of course, is a strong argument against using excessive quantities of cold, draining medicines that drain replete fire. There is a fine distinction necessary between dispelling replete fire evils and draining essential fire stored in the right kidneys (*mìng mén* 命門/life gate). This is not only a problem in modern traditional Chinese medicine practice, which often mimics modern medicine's use of cold, draining pharmaceuticals such as antibiotics and anti-inflammatories, but in modern

---

2   Unschuld and Tessenow 2011: 743

medical practice in general. Heat/fire evils in general are often misdiagnosed when what is truly occurring is that the body's vital heat sources, expressed through *xiàng huǒ* 相火/ministerial fire and *wèi qì* 衛氣/defense *qì*, are attempting to dispel evil cold, not heat.

In the commentaries on *Nàn Jīng* 難經 8, we find profound discussions on ministerial fire (*xiàng huǒ* 相火). According to Lǚ Guǎng 呂廣, "the triple burner distributes the *yíng qì* 營氣 and the *wèi qì* 衛氣, and it bars *xié qì* 邪氣/evil qì from entering at will."[3] Yè Lín 葉霖 states:

> the moving *qi* between the kidneys are the original of the vital *qì* of the twelve jing/conduit vessels, they control the *yíng qì* 營氣 and the *wèi qì* 衛氣. The moving up and down of the *qì* and blood in the human body depends on exhalation and inhalation to maintain their circulation. Through inhalation the *yáng qì* of heaven enter; through exhalation the *yīn qì* of the earth leave the body. Fire is transformed into *qì* when brought into water.[4]

Yè Lín 葉霖 is describing the dragon fire that resides within the water phase of the kidney, which then transforms into vital *qì*. Lǐ Jiǒng 李駉 goes on to describe the movement of the *qì* in the *chōng mài* 衝脈/thoroughway vessel emerging from between the kidneys.

We see again the importance of breath and its connection with vessel dynamics, the root of the *sān jiāo* 三膲 and *chōng mài* 衝脈 in ministerial fire (*xiàng huǒ* 相火)/*mìng mén* 命門, and the basis of the interactions of defense and construction *qì*, the descent of heavenly fire from the heart via the *dū mài* 督脈/governor vessel to the kidneys, the transformation of water by bladder *qì*, which steams upwards to form sweat.

Wáng Hào-gǔ 王好古 sums all of this up as follows in his discussion on the *chōng mài* 衝脈:

---

3 Unschuld (Nán Jīng) 2016: 108
4 ibid: 109

the *shào yáng* 少陽 *sān jiāo* 三膲 is one dwelling place of the ministerial fire, the right kidney life gate is the ministerial fire, and the *xīn bāo* 心包/heart envelope master is also called the ministerial fire. These vessels are all diagnosed in the same manner. The kidney is the gate of *qì* generation. It emerges from and governs the area below the umbilicus, and it is divided into three forks surging upward through the umbilicus via St. 25 (*tiān shū* 天樞), ascending to reach CV 17 (*shān zhōng* 膻中) beside both breasts. This is where the primal *qì* is tied in.[5]

In *Nàn Jīng* 難經 66, it says that "the *qì* moving below the navel and between the kidneys constitutes man's life. They are the source and basis of the twelve (main) channels. The *sān jiāo* 三焦/triple burner is the special envoy that transmits the *yuán qì* 原氣/original *qì*." This *qì* can be accessed at *yuán* 原 points discussed in *Nàn Jīng* 難經 5.

In *Nán Jīng* 難經 24, the specific diagnostic signs and symptoms are listed to inform us which of the six paired *yīn/yáng* channels have been severed from *yuán qì* 原氣 and *xiàng huǒ* 相火/ministerial fire, as in these scenarios, since the vessel qualities sometimes doesn't reflect the internal condition. In these cases, it is like seeing the light in the firmament from distant stars that died millions of years ago, but is still being viewed from earth.

II. Difficult Issue 24 discusses the principle in Chinese medicine known as *zàng xiàng* 臟象/visceral manifestation. This is a fundamental concept in Chinese medicine, based on 1) the intimate connection of the viscera and bowels with their associated channels and 2) the relationship of external signs associated with the tissues and sense organs with their internal viscera and bowels.

The relationships are as follows:

- The foot *shào yīn* 少陰 channel warms the marrow and the bones. When the *shào yīn* 少陰 channel fails to

---

5   Chace, Shima, and Li 2010: 27

communicate with the kidneys, the bones wither, the flesh becomes loose on the bones, softens, and shrinks. The teeth become long and wither, hair loses its glossiness and moisture.

- The foot *tài yīn* 太陰 channel, when cut off, no long supplies the mouth and lips with *qì*. They represent the foundation of the flesh/*ròu* 肉. The flesh is no longer smooth and moist, the lips curl back and the flesh dies on days associated with the wood phase.

- The foot *jué yīn* 厥陰 channel nourishes the *jīn* 筋/sinews. When the channel communication is severed, the testicles shrink and the tongue rolls back.

- The hand *tài yīn* 太陰 channel nourishes the skin and body hair. When the channel is severed, the skin and body hair will be scorched, the liquids depart, the skin and joints are harmed, the skin withers and the hair breaks off.

- The hand *shào yīn* 少陰 channel governs the blood vessels. When the channel is severed, the blood cannot flow, the complexion and glossiness fade, and there is a black complexion indicating death of the blood.

- When the three *yīn* vessels are all severed, vision becomes dizzy, the eyes remain closed or lose control, one loses one's mind, and the mind eventually dies.

- When the three *yáng* vessels are cut off, the *yīn* and *yáng* aspects of the organism are separated from each other. The pores are drained, there is intermittent sweat like a string of pearls without flow. This means that the *qì* has expired. If it occurs in the morning, one dies at night. If at night, one dies the next morning.

We see that there are correspondences with the tissue, channel, sense organs, and the days of the Chinese calendar that are associated with each channel. This chapter completes the concepts in *Nàn Jīng* 難經 Difficult Issue 9 (*Severance of the Vessels*) of the situation where the kidney *qi*'s decline is not visible in the movement of the vessels.

What do we mean by severance of the vessels? The channels no longer communicate with the viscera, bowels, and their associated tissues and sense organs. This is of extreme importance in the medicine of the *Nàn Jīng* 難經. Health is seen to be free-flowing communication of the channels between all associated structures and functions, emotions and behaviors. The channels establish communication and homeostasis within the body and they must be synchronized with the external environment with its multitude of interactive rhythms and cycles. Acupuncture, as described in the *Nàn Jīng* 難經, is designed to correct, restore, and maintain this homeostasis, based on the judgment of the physician through careful diagnosis and treatment. The symptoms described in this chapter are based on a logical order and series of correspondences, where one can trace a person's movements towards life or death and prognosis.

CHAPTER 8

NÁN JĪNG 難經 9

Distinguishing Rapid and Slow Vessel Movements in Relationship to Viscera and Bowels

In Difficult Issue 9, we further differentiate the vessel dynamics via *yīn* and *yáng*, through examining the speed of the vessel movements. Here, diseases of the *zàng* 臟/*yīn* viscera are indicated by slow vessel movements. A rapid or quick vessel movement indicates illness in the *fǔ* 腑/bowels. All authorities agree a more rapid vessel movement is associated with heat, causing a stirring (*dòng* 動) of the vessels, whereas, all slowness of vessel movements indicates cold. *Yáng* symptoms are replete heat, as in *yáng míng bing* 陽明病 in the *Shāng Hán Lùn* 傷寒論, and *yīn* symptoms are cold such as *shāng hán* 傷寒/cold damage in the *Shāng Hán Lùn* 傷寒論. If we see rapid movements in the vessels, it indicates that the *yáng qì* is being stirred. If we see slow vessel movements, the *yīn* viscera are being affected and this is consistent with what the *Shāng Hán Lùn* 傷寒論 teaches us in terms of interior/exterior disease, three *yáng* channel diseases, and three *yīn* channel diseases. There is no conflict here.

So, to the *yīn*/*yáng* differentiation of interior/exterior, *cùn* 寸/inch and *chǐ* 尺/cubit (foot) vessels, we now add speed of vessel movement to further broaden the logical system on which vessel dynamics are constructed in the *Nán Jīng* 難經.

CHAPTER 9

NÀN JĪNG 難經 10
The Wǔ Xié 五邪/Five Evils and Ten Variations

In describing *xié qì* 邪氣/evil *qì* in the *Sù Wèn* 素問, Paul Unschuld has indicated that 邪 xie/evil means any phenomena that has violated its normal place in the scheme of nature, based on the ideal of Confucian society. Acupuncture treatment was designed in the *Sù Wèn* 素問, to "repair the walls before the thief enters."[1] The same chapter also teaches that "where *xié qì* 邪氣/evil *qì* collects, the *zhèng qì* 正氣/correct *qì* must be depleted." In *Sù Wèn* 素問 68, it says, "where there is correspondence, then there is compliance. If not so, there is opposition. Where there is opposition, then this gives rise to changes.[2] Where there are changes, then there is disease."[3]

In his version of the *Nàn Jīng* 難經, Paul describes five evils that can afflict the *zàng fǔ* 臟腑 if they violate each other. The first is *zhèng xié* 正邪/correct evil, where a viscera or bowel falls ill by itself. The next is *xū xié* 虛邪/vacuity evil, where the mother phase attacks the child phase, as if from behind. Next is a *shí xié* 實邪/repletion evil, where the child phase attacks the mother, from ahead. Next is *wēi xié* 微邪/weakness evil, when the evil is transmitted backwards from the controlled phase

---

1   Unschuld 2003
2   *biàn* 變/change (*dòng* 動/stirring)
3   Unschuld and Tessenow 2011: 218

(for example, the lungs/metal are controlled by the heart/fire) by the controlling cycle that skips phases. Finally is a *zéi xié* 賊邪/ destroyer (thief) evil, where the controlling phase transmits the disease to the controlled phase (the heart/fire transmits the disease to the lung/metal).

One of the most interesting aspects of *Nàn Jīng* 難經 vessel diagnosis is feeling five phase relationships within the positions in terms of specific qualities. In other words, we can feel wiry qualities in the metal/*tài yīn* 太陰 position, hair-like qualities in the wood/*jué yīn* 厥陰 position. The specific vessel qualities discussed in Difficult Issues 15 and 16 are here shown as relational to specific disease patterns, seasons, and behavior. Qualities associated with specific channels and viscera/bowels are now seen to be signs of disease when appearing in positions associated with other channels, viscera/bowels, and qualities. It is a form of "disassociation" of qualities appearing where they should not. This is consistent with the general tendency in Chinese medicine for qualities to belong to certain phases and stages, in a certain progression through time and space. When these changes happen in an orderly manner, health and equilibrium are maintained. When the normal cycles of visceral function are disturbed, disease results.

The *Nàn Jīng* 難經 has developed a model of homeostasis that could be appreciated by an endocrinologist or immunologist practicing today. The text provides several models for observing the flow of change in the human being, and treatment strategies to correct the loss of equilibrium with the self, time, and the environment.

In the *Nàn Jīng* 難經, evils are not necessarily seen as being contracted from the exterior, but within the viscera and bowels themselves, and transmitted via the five phase cycle between each other. The root concept here is that any excessive influence from a viscera or bowel that "overflows" its area of influence, or any vacuity of a viscera or bowel (or its associated channel) is "evil" in and of itself. The balanced, normal functioning of the visceral systems is disturbed, leading to disease. As Katō Bankei, a Japanese commentator on the *Nàn Jīng* 難經 states, each section of the movement in the vessels (*cùn guān chǐ* 寸關尺/ inch, bar, cubit) may show that the *qì* of one channel, viscera, or bowel may "invade" or enter another position, causing disease.

Diseased vessel movements may indicate that the *qì* of one phase may "escape" and appear in another phase. This means that one finds the quality (wiry, relaxed, replete, vacuous, soft) associated with a phase in a position associated with another phase. For example, sometimes the middle position on the right wrist will be wiry, while it will be relaxed on the left wrist in the middle position. This means that liver *qì* has violated the spleen, and has "vacated" its normal position. If the left-hand middle position is vacuous or soft, this is often a sign of severe liver disease. The *Nàn Jīng* 難經 teaches that one has to "recover" the *qì* and bring it back to its original position with acupuncture treatment, using the five transporting points on each channel. This situation may also be affected by *shí qì* 時氣/seasonal *qì*. In other words, liver *qì* tends to be more replete in the spring time, so a wiry vessel quality in summer time in the heart position means that *xié qì* 邪氣/evil *qì* from the liver has attacked the heart. While this text is focused on vessel diagnosis, and not on acupuncture/moxibustion treatment strategies, the treatment section of the *Nàn Jīng* 難經 explains this methodology in depth.

CHAPTER 10

NÁN JĪNG 難經 11
Arrival and Departure of Qi in the Wǔ Zàng 五臟/Five Yīn Viscera

Líng Shū 靈樞 Chapter 5 (*Gēn Jié*/根結 *Root and Connection*), discusses that during one day and one night the *wèi qì* 衛氣 and *yíng qì* 營氣 pass through 50 cycles, and in this way they supply the five *zàng* 臟 with essence. The first Difficult Issue of the *Nán Jīng* 難經 also builds on this particular circulation of *yíng* 營/*wèi* 衛 as the rationale for focusing on the *cùn kǒu* 寸口/ inch mouth location for reading vessel dynamics.

Here we see the 24-hour cycle of *wèi qì* 衛氣/defense *qì* and *yíng qì* 營氣/construction *qì* illustrated in the regularity of the vessels, which reflect the internal state of the *wǔ zàng* 五臟/five viscera. As the *qì* moves six *cùn* 寸 with each inhalation and exhalation through the channels as described in Difficult Issue 1of the *Nàn Jīng* 難經, at nighttime it penetrates the *wǔ zàng* 五臟/viscera to nourish the *yuán qì* 元氣/original *qì* of each viscus. If this circulation is not smooth, then the movement in the vessel stops and starts, with feelings of obstruction or actual missed beats. From this chapter, we can see the importance of regular activity during the day and rest at night. When activity and rest/sleep are disturbed, the viscera do not receive nourishment, and the following day when the sun rises, the person feels exhaustion from depletion of the kidneys. In modern culture, where circadian rhythms are greatly disturbed by staying up late, over-stimulation from light sources, travel, noise, and entertainment, many people find it difficult to compensate for this morning exhaustion (the time of the greatest *yáng qì* potential) and wake up very tired and unable to think clearly. This leads to an almost universal dependence on caffeine to function, and to "drag oneself out of bed." However, the reliance on caffeine only exacerbates kidney depletion, and eventually the person gets ill or ages prematurely in an attempt for the body/mind to replenish itself in the rest that was lost, with symptoms such as hearing loss, tinnitus, hair loss, impotence, urinary difficulty, or vaginal dryness.

Many of my patients suffer from this kidney depletion, and rely on compensation strategies to function on a day-to-day basis, such as sleeping in on weekends. This will only further throw off the natural circadian rhythms, and as the person gets older, this strategy will not work as well. In these patients, the movement in the vessels will either be deep, faint, or irregular, or if caffeinated, flooding and/or rapid without root. This will be accompanied by a low, groaning voice and grayish complexion.

Nán Jīng 難經 Difficulty 11 establishes that inhaled *qì* are associated with *yáng*, and enter via the *zàng* 臟/*yīn* viscera. Exhaled *qì* are associated with *yīn*, and exit through the *fǔ* 腑/*yáng* bowels. According to Lǐ Jiǒng 李駉, inhaled *qì* enters the liver and kidneys below the diaphragm (*yīn* portion, lower body), while exhaled *qì* exists through the heart and lung above the diaphragm (*yáng* portion, upper body). But when the rhythms of *yīn* and *yáng* are disturbed, by not living with the *qì* of the season, time of day, circadian rhythms, rest and activity, the inhaled *qì* may reach the liver, but bypass the kidneys. Hence, the *yuán qì* 原氣/original *qì* received from one's parents (constitutional *jīng* 精/essence) becomes depleted. We see Huá Shòu 滑壽 make a similar commentary, stating:

Of the five *yīn* viscera, the kidneys are located lowest; they are the most distant viscus to be reached by the inhaled *qì*. If the movement stops in less than fifty arrivals, one knows that the kidneys do not receive any supplies; their *qì* will be depleted first. *Jìn* 盡 "depleted" means *shuāi jié* 衰竭 "exhausted." If they are exhausted, they cannot follow the *qì* of the other *yīn* viscera and move upward.[1]

---

1   Unschuld (*Nán Jīng*) 2016: 132

CHAPTER 11

NÁN JĪNG 難經 14

Injury and Arrival in the Movement in the Vessels

The way to understand *sǔn* 損/injury or *zhì* 至/arrival is in terms of circadian rhythms. In other words, the *wèi qì* 衛氣/defense *qì* descends into the five *yīn* viscera at nighttime, arriving in the kidneys before dawn, before reversing outwards towards the exterior as the *yáng qì* increases. This cycle also connects with the breathing rhythm and sleep schedule disturbances such as lost or disturbed sleep, and rapid or depleted breathing will be seen in the vessel rhythm. If the kidneys do not receive the *qì*, the person will feel exhausted the following day. The speeding up of the vessels or breathing rhythms (via activity, heat, cold, season, evil *qì*), or slowing down, has a profound effect on the *wǔ zàng* 五藏/five *yīn* viscera. Sleep, waking, and activity cycles all must be regulated, along with the breath, in order to maintain health. In the five stages of *sǔn* 損/injury, the various *yīn* viscera and associated tissues are *shāng* 傷/damaged. We see this explained in Dīng Dé-yòng's 丁德用 commentary that:

> when the spleen is injured, one must balance the intake of food and drink, and provide the appropriate amounts of cold and heat. It is said that the spleen controls *sī* 思/thought and intellect. Hence, one must bring the intellect, and thought, as well as his food and drink, into compliance.[1]

---

1 Unschuld (*Nán Jīng*) 2016: 163

In each stage of *sǔn* 損/injury, the tissue associated with each viscus shows signs of damage. In the first stage (lung viscus), there is injury of skin and body hair. In the second stage, the *mài* 脈/vessels (associated with the heart) lack blood and essence to circulate through the body. In the third stage, the *ròu* 肉/flesh associated with the spleen is injured, leading to emaciation and inability to assimilate. In the fourth stage, the muscles associated with the liver relax and cannot support the skeletal structure. In the fifth and final stage, the bones associated with the kidneys are injured, and one cannot rise out of bed. This is a movement from the exterior to the interior. However, an illness can also be generated outwards from interior to exterior with the final stage as injury to skin and body hair (see Figure 11.1). Each stage of injury has a treatment strategy. For lung/metal damage, supplement the *qì*. For the heart, balance *wèi qì* 衛氣 and *yíng qì* 營氣. For spleen, balance food and drink, and exposure to heat and cold. For the liver, relax the *zhōng* 中/center. For the kidneys, supplement the *jīng* 精/essence. Each of these treatment strategies can be implemented with needle or moxa therapy, herbal medicine, diet, exercises, breathing practice, or lifestyle changes.

The text then continues with a discussion of vessel dynamics corresponding to inhalation and exhalation, specifically the speed of vessel movements during one in-breath and out-breath, strong or weak *cùn* 寸 and *chǐ* 尺 vessels. With *sǔn* 損/injury from exterior to interior, illnesses descend from the lungs to the kidneys, with a weakening speed of movement in the vessels. Illness can also ascend from the kidneys to the exterior, with increasing strength and frequency; this is called *zhì* 至/arrival. Katō Bankei points out in his commentary that, "*zhì* 至/arriving stands for *jìn* 近/approaching. *Sǔn* 損/injured stands for *tuì* 退/withdrawing."[2] So, unification occurs with the in-breath, separation with the out-breath. This can be tracked to follow the course of illness in our patients.

---

2   Unschuld (*Nán Jīng*) 2016: 155

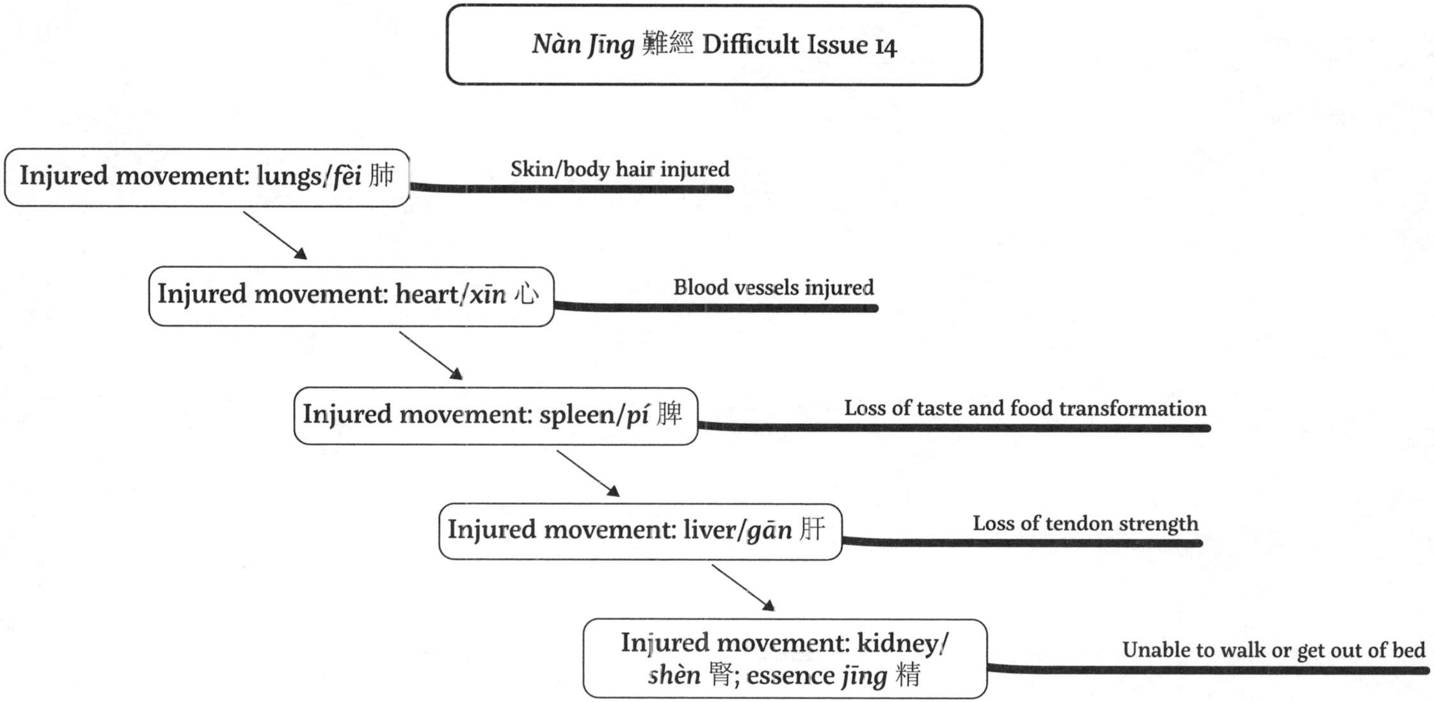

Nàn Jīng 難經 Difficult Issue 14

Skin/body hair injured

Injured movement: lungs/*fèi* 肺

Blood vessels injured

Injured movement: heart/*xīn* 心

Loss of taste and food transformation

Injured movement: spleen/*pí* 脾

Loss of tendon strength

Injured movement: liver/*gān* 肝

Unable to walk or get out of bed

Injured movement: kidney/*shèn* 腎; essence *jīng* 精

Figure 11.1: Nàn Jīng 難經 *Difficult Issue 14*

CHAPTER 12

NÀN JĪNG 難經 15 VISCERAL MOVEMENTS IN THE VESSELS

Reading Qualities of Amplitude

Difficult Issue 15 of the *Nàn Jīng* 難經 explains the seasonal vessel movements illustrating that it is essential that modern practitioners sensitize themselves to the rhythms of nature. The human being is a very sensitive instrument of flesh and conscious awareness that responds to very subtle signals and changes in the environment. The time of year, the angle of sunlight, the length of day and night, lunar changes, and planetary/orbital positions influence the human organism. These can all be read in vessel dynamics as an important key to pathological changes that are going on with the patient, allowing the physician to read both global and local influences to health. In order to do this, practitioners needs to sensitize themselves to these rhythms so that they know how to recognize them and how to read them. One of the most fascinating things about vessel dynamics that I have observed in my practice is that before there are weather changes, the body is already responding with changes in the vessel movements with associated symptoms. Most *shāng hán* 傷寒/cold damage invasion-type epidemics occur within days before major weather changes, which can be observed in vessel dynamics.

There are normal seasonal vessel movements, but there are also exaggerated seasonal movements. In other words, all the seasonal movements in the vessels are modified by the presence of spleen stomach *qì*, which gives a suppleness and balance and a quality of earth *qì* to the vessels. When a viscera is diseased, the quality will become harsh like the wiry quality associated with spring time, and excessive liver *qì* becomes overly exuberant. So, the practitioner has to read the amplitude of the vessel quality as well as the seasonal quality. This tells you something about disease and that the visceral system is attempting to compensate. Related viscera according to the operating principles of *wǔ xíng* 五行/five phase dynamics are compensating for repletion and depletions which will generally will lead to a disease state or pattern of disharmony. On examining the kidney vessel movements, I have observed that when the vessel quality is sinking and stone-like, it will feel exaggerated like a hard ball of rubber bands with a very uneven form and shape. You literally can feel the *jīng* 精/essence of the kidney desiccating. Lǎo Zǐ 老子 says that life is supple and flexible and responds to change, and death is hard and inflexible and breaks. This is the same with the vessel dynamics associated with the seasonal vessel movements. The suppleness is the sign of life and even if there is disharmony or disease, the flexibility of the body will help to restore homeostasis. However, if the body is hardened, exaggerated, and inflexible, it may be much more difficult to bring the person back to health. In the aging process, often the movement in the vessels becomes obstructed, occluded, or hardened and, in this case, we need to focus on restoring suppleness and grace to the vessel dynamic.

Nàn Jīng 難經 15 is also based on discussions outlined in Sù Wèn 素問 18 and 19. In Sù Wèn 素問 18, it is said that "the regular *qì* of a normal person is supplied by the stomach. When someone has no stomach *qì*, that is called contrary movement."[1] In Zhāng Zhì-cong's 張志聰 commentary, he points out that "the movement in the vessels of the *wǔ zàng* 五臟/five *yīn* viscera

---

1   Unschuld and Tessenow 2011: 303

depends on the stomach."[2] If *yíng qì* 營氣 produced by the stomach does not circulate to a viscus, that viscus will atrophy and "die." While the person may continue to live, it will be in a highly biased fashion, or the viscus will acquire a serious disease, such as an autoimmune disorder (autoimmune hepatitis, for example). At the very least, biasing will occur and the functions of one viscus will be shunted to another viscus in an attempt to compensate. This is not dissimilar to the dynamics of a dysfunctional family, where dysfunctional family members are compensated for by other family members who "fill in the gaps" (as with children of alcoholics).

In *Sù Wèn* 素問 19, a specific *zàng* 臟/visceral movement in the vessels is described as being without *wèi qì* 衛氣. When there is a *zhēn zàng mài* 真臟脈/genuine visceral movement in the vessels, it indicates that the viscus is "running on empty," and must expire at some point. For example, many patients with kidney disease will have a harsh, "rocky" vessel quality. This feels like hard pebbles, rather than smooth and stone-like. This vessel quality is often visible in patients who are suffering from kidney failure or who are on dialysis. The reason why this is called "genuine vessel movement" is that when you feel a strong, exaggerated vessel quality without stomach *qì*, it means that the vessel is in a hyperactive state, indicating a "last gasp" of the body in maintaining visceral function.

The movement in the vessels can be amplified or diminished, depending on the *biàn huà* 變化. Sabine Wilms describes in her book *Humming with Elephants: The Great Treatise on the Resonant Manifestations of Yīn and Yáng* that:

> The phrase *biàn huà* 變化 which simply means "change" in modern Chinese, is actually a reference to two specific types of change. Huà 化 describes sudden, irreversible, substantive, and often generative change, in the literal sense of "metamorphosis"

---

2   Unschuld and Tessenow 2011: 307

such as from a pupa to the butterfly, or from non-being to being. *Biàn* 變, on the other hand, refers to gradual, slow alterations such as between yīn yáng, night and day, water and ice or seasonal changes.[3]

This determines the condition of the viscera associated with its season. But all of the seasonal vessel qualities gain their suppleness, pliability, and liveliness from the stomach *qì*, which provides *yíng qì* 營氣. Without this, the movement in the vessels is harsh, like old, dry, dead wood.

Before establishing the movement of the vessels in disease, we must first establish the movements of the vessels in normal health, relative to a patient's constitution. This includes the time of day, and season, while taking into account the various vessel influences delineated in Appendix 1. The "perfect" movement in the vessels can be described as a "sine wave," with equal rise and fall, and a smooth, harmonious quality which in *Nàn Jīng* 難經 15 is described as containing stomach *qì*. The normal heart vessel qualities is described in *Sù Wèn* 素問 18 as "strung together, resembling a string of pearls; if feels as if one's fingers passed over *láng gān* 琅玕/jade like stone."[4] Other examples of the centrality of the earth phase include the following: 1) the *tài yīn* 太陰 phase in the *Shāng Hán Lùn* 傷寒論 and the inclusion of spleen-supplementing herbs in a large percentage of formulas in the text; 2) the last 18 days of each season correspond to earth and spleen/stomach *qì*; 3) Lǐ Dōng-yuán's 李東垣 spleen/stomach current *Bǔ Tǔ Pài* 補土派; emphasizing that earth is the central phase around which the other phases circle. Stomach *qì* modifies the more extreme characteristics of each phase exhibited in the vessel movements, and its decline or depletion leads to exaggerated qualities in the resulting vessel image.

The stomach is the sea of water and grains; it is responsible for supplying the five yīn viscera during all four seasons. Hence,

---

3   Wilms 2018: 28
4   Unschuld and Tessenow 2011: 318

the stomach *qì* is the basis for them. This is what is meant by variations in the movement of the vessels and by disease related to the four seasons; these are the essential criteria for recognizing a person's impending death or survival. The spleen is the central region; when balanced and in its normal state it cannot be recognized through feeling the movement in the vessels. Only in its exhaustion can it be recognized. In this case, the movement in the vessels arrives like the pecking of birds, like the dripping of water. This is how one can recognize exhaustion of the spleen.

CHAPTER 13

NÁN JĪNG 難經 13 AND 16

Explanation of Corresponding
Internal/External Evidence
with Vessel Discrimination

Nán Jīng 難經 13 presents an innovative diagnostic and treatment strategy, tying together vessel movement and complexion, correspondences together described in *Líng Shū* 靈樞 4. Figure 13.1 below compares the two chapters. *Nán Jīng* 難經 13, after comparing the *sè* 色/complexion, with the *mài* 脈/vessel, then develops a five phase treatment system based on these correspondences of the *shēng* 生 and *kè* 剋 cycles. The text demonstrates when vessel dynamics and complexion correspond, when they do not, and how that is expressed in terms of diagnosis and prognosis, some of which according to the text can be critical. Reading and diagnosing *sè* 色/complexion is described in detail in several chapters of the *Líng Shū* 靈樞, including Chapter 4, The Physical Appearances of Diseases and Chapter 49, Five Complexions (*wǔ sè* 五色), explaining that each color and complexion corresponds to a specific part of the face.

In the *Sù Wèn* 素問, the spleen region corresponds to the area around the lips. The kidney corresponds to the area around the chin, the lung region above the eyebrows, the heart region around the mouth, the liver region below the eyes. Various relationships of the colors/complexions are described in terms of five phase theory, such as colors in the wrong location, the area of the face sunken in, the size of the colored area—in other words, this is a fairly complex diagnostic system. Here the *Nán Jīng* 難經 limits itself to comparing vessel dynamics with complexion as a specific diagnostic system. This is yet another area of Chinese medicine diagnostics that is largely under-utilized in modern practice, yet valuable to the point that the *Líng Shū* 靈樞 states that a superior practitioner utilizes questioning, vessel dynamics and complexion in one's diagnosis. As we discussed earlier in the text, vessel dynamics were never meant to be practiced in isolation, but in congruence with questioning, palpating the vessels at large and the abdomen, and viewing changes to the face and skin. This included temperature, moisture, tension, tone, smoothness (or rough areas), along with sound of voice, shape and size of sense organs, viewing hands, shapes of fingers and toes, odors, and expression of emotions and personality. All of these signs and symptoms, taken in *yìng* 應/resonance, gave a complete picture to the physician and allowed for a comprehensive diagnosis based on *zàng xiàng* 臟象/visceral manifestation.[1]

We see in the *Sù Wèn* 素問 17 that the movement in the vessel is the moon and the complexion is the sun, and that together vessel and complexion are essential to each other. *Sè* 色/complexion is described by Wáng Bīng 王冰 as the "sun" to the "moon" of *mài zhěn* 脈診/vessel examination in chapter 3 of the *Sù Wèn* 素問,[2] and to be used in resonance with it.

However, in modern practice, complexion is not used widely, much less so than vessel diagnosis, which in and of itself has lost much prominence in the modern practice of traditional Chinese medicine. I find, in chronic, serious illnesses, and occasionally in acute disorders, especially in children, that these colors can be outstanding. For example, the blackish color under the eyes indicating kidney depletion or poor sleep is very common, as are red cheeks in children with respiratory issues. Spleen vacuity

---

1   This is discussed in depth in my first book *Returning to the Source: Han Dynasty Medical Classics in Modern Clinical Practice* (2018)

2   Unschuld and Tessenow 2011: 224

patients often have a yellowish, sallow complexion. I tend to corroborate vessel diagnosis along with tongue diagnosis, which is a much later development in Chinese medical history.[3]

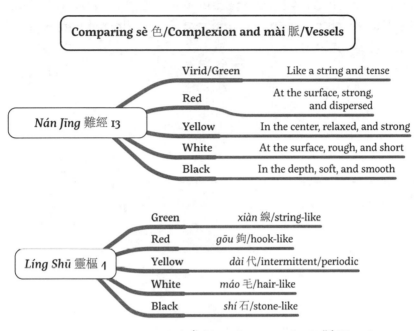

Figure 13.1: Comparing sè 色/Complexion and mài 脈/Vessels

Nán Jīng 難經 16 gives us additional confirmation diagnostics that correspond with vessel dynamics. *Nán Jīng* 難經 Difficult Issue 16 includes abdominal palpation, setting the foundation for all future abdominal palpation methods developed by Japanese physicians, specifically the foundational work of Tōdō Yoshimasu 吉益東洞, an 18th-century physician who relied almost entirely on abdominal palpation for diagnosis. Sometimes vessel dynamics will give us sufficient information to get a definitive diagnosis, but in many cases, because of medications, damage to the wrist, or bifurcation of the wrist vessels, it may not be possible to rely just on the *cùn kǒu* 寸口. In these cases,

---

3 For an excellent translation of two tongue diagnosis texts see *Gold Mirrors and Tongue Reflections: The Cornerstone Classics of Chinese Medicine Tongue Diagnosis* (Solos 2012)

the physician can utilize specific channel system vessels in other parts of the body. I will often palpate KI 3 (*tài xī* 太谿), LR 3 (*tài chōng* 太沖), ST 30 (*qì chōng* 氣衝), *tài yáng* 太陽 and so on, and especially ST 42 (*chōng yáng* 衝陽). In the *Shāng Hán Lùn* 傷寒論, this is called the *fū yáng mài* 趺陽脈/instep *yáng* vessel.

CHAPTER 14

NÀN JĪNG 難經 18

The Core Vessel Dynamics Maps of the Nàn Jīng 難經

The *Nàn Jīng* 難經 integrates channel theory with *zàng fǔ* 臟腑/visceral/bowel theory, five phase theory with *yīn* and *yáng* methods of diagnosis. This is no more apparent than in Difficult Issue 18, a discussion of the information contained in each of the three divisions of the movements in the vessel: *cùn guān chǐ* 寸關尺/inch, bar, and cubit as it pertains to the channels and contents of upper, middle, and lower burners respectively.

What is extraordinary in this discussion is that it seamlessly integrates information from both an *jīng luò* 經絡 acupuncture/channel-connecting vessel perspective, and an internal medicine *zàng fǔ* 臟腑 viscera/bowel perspective in one vessel dynamics map. Here we see the basis for applying palpation of the vessels to treatment by acumoxa therapy, and as the basis for the major part of vessel diagnosis in Japanese acupuncture, and even the J.R. Worsley system of five element acupuncture. One can observe qualities of the paired channels and their five phase relationships, and use the five transporting points (*wǔ shū xué* 五輸穴) to balance the *jīng luò* 經絡 channels and network vessels. The flow of *qì* from left to right, one side of the body to the other, resembles a figure of eight, following the dynamics of the channels and five phase transformations (see Figure 14.1).

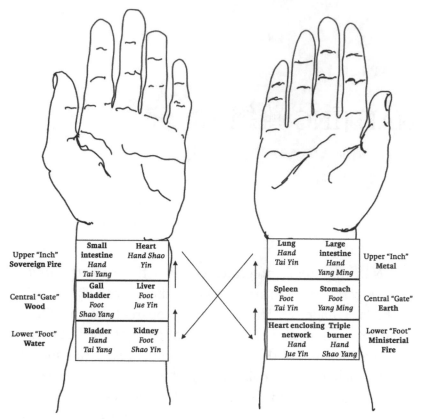

Figure 14.1: Nán Jīng 難經 *18 Vessel Diagram*

The next section of Difficult Issue 18, however, takes an alternative perspective on palpating the vessels:

脈有三部九候，各何所主之？

The movement in the vessels appears in three sections and on nine indicator (levels). By which illnesses are the (movements in these sections and on these levels) governed, respectively?

然：三部者，寸，關，尺也。九候者，浮、中、沉也。上部法天，主胸以上至頭之有疾也；中部法人，主膈以下至齊之有疾也；下部法地，主齊以下至足之有疾也。審而刺之者也。

It is like this. The three sections concerned are inch, bar, and cubit. The nine indicator levels refer to surface, center and depth (of each section). The upper section is patterned on heaven; it is governed by illnesses located from the chest upward to the head. The central section is patterned after man; it is governed by illnesses located below the diaphragm to the navel. The lower section is patterned after earth; it is governed by illnesses located below the navel to the feet.[1]

In this section, we see a more internal, viscera-bowel oriented approach to vessel dynamics, similar to the orientation of Lǐ Shízhēn's 李時珍 *Bīn Hú Mài Xué* 瀕湖脈學/*Lakeside Master's Pulse Study* (17th century). At this point, we need to ask, what is the difference between *jīng luò* 經絡 channel/connecting vessel and *zàng fǔ* 臟腑/viscera/bowel pattern differentiation? The former applies more to acupuncture/moxibustion treatment, the latter to internal medicine (treatment by Chinese medicinals). With the channels and *luò mài* 絡脈/network vessels, we are concentrating on the informational system that connects all parts of the body, flowing dynamically between the *yīn* interior region and *yáng* exterior region of the body. The channel system responds quickly to change, constantly readjusting the flow of *qì* to maintain systemic equilibrium. The channel system connects with the interior via the connecting vessels and *bié mài* 別脈/divergent channels, allowing the *zàng* 臟/viscera and *fǔ* 腑/bowels to send information to the exterior, and respond to external stimuli. Being more dense and substantial, the viscera and bowels move and respond more slowly than the channels. In severe disorders, the connection between the viscera/bowels and the channels may be severed, as discussed in Difficult Issue 24. This loss of communication is often behind many serious disorders, especially damage to the associated tissues of the five viscera.

The *sān jiāo* 三膲/three burners are divided among the *cùn guān chǐ* 寸關尺 inch, bar, and foot/cubit, and their contents can be palpated in great detail. Within each position, one can palpate the condition of *qì*, blood and fluids, viscera and bowels, using the

---

1   Unschuld (*Nán Jīng*) 2016: 206

28 vessel qualities enumerated in the *Mài Jīng* 脈經/*Pulse Classic* to determine the qualities of disease patterns. The upper burner, as discussed in Difficult Issue 31, is treated at Ren 17(*shān zhōng* 膻中), and governs transformation of *dà qì* 大氣/great *qì* or air *qì*. The middle burner, treated at St 25 (*tiān shū* 天樞), governs transformation of food and drink, and separation of clear and turbid. The lower burner, treated at Ren 5 (*shí mén* 石門) or 6 (*qì hǎi* 氣海), governs transformation and separation of fluids.

The final section of *Nàn Jīng* 難經 18 (lines 12–19) discusses the effects of *jī* 積/accumulations and blockages on vessel qualities: *zhì* 滯/knotted (stagnant) and *chén* 沉/ sunken; deep. Line 17 tells us that *chén* 沉/subdued means that the movement in the vessels occurs below the muscles (mid-level). At the surface means that the movement in the vessels occurs above the flesh. *Jié mài* 結脈/ bound vessel is a vessel that is moderate or slow and pauses at irregular intervals. The *Mài Jīng* 脈經 states that it "indicates exuberant *yīn* and bound *qì* , congested *qì* and stagnant phlegm, or concretions, conglomerations accumulations and gatherings"[2]

In clinical practice, one of the most critical aspects of my diagnosis is finding accumulations of *qì*, phlegm, and static blood in different regions in the body, the *jīng luò* 經絡, or in the *zàng fǔ* 臟腑/viscera/bowels and their associated tissues. Since this is so common in modern patients, due to sedentary lifestyle, poor diet, stress, climate, age, and constitutional factors, having these tools of vessel diagnosis which can then be translated into treatment strategies is essential. For clinical cases, please see Chapter 18, which includes case histories.

---

2   Wiseman and Ye 1998: 48

CHAPTER 15

NÁN JĪNG 難經 20

Discussing the Yīn Yáng Aspects of Vessels in Appropriate Vessel Qualities Being Hidden and Concealed

Difficult Issue 20 is similar to what we discussed in Chapter 3 with *Nán Jīng* 難經 2 and 3, in terms of distinguishing *yīn* vessels from *yáng* vessels. *Yáng* vessels normally have their domain in the *cùn* 寸 position and *yīn* vessels have their domain in the *chǐ* 尺 foot position, with the *guān* 關 as the bar or gate separating the two, between *yīn* and *yáng* on the vessels. We also established that *yáng* vessels are at the exterior with light (finger) pressure and that *yīn* are in the interior domain with stronger pressure.

Now, in Difficult Issue 20, we are discussing when *yīn qì* 陰氣 is found in the *yáng* position i.e. the exterior, and *yáng qì* 陽氣 is found in the interior, in the *yīn* section. Here, *yīn* and *yáng* have reversed each other qualitatively and in terms of their correct location. In the *Nán Jīng* 難經, everything has its correct place and order, in heaven and earth, in nature and in humanity; this is a Confucian view of the world. In terms of the five phases, each phases has a vessel dynamic that is correct, and each season has a vessel dynamic that is normally associated with it. When a vessel quality is found in the five phase visceral dynamic outside its normal location, as when a wiry vessel dynamic is found in the earth right *guān* 關 position and is replete, while the left *guān* 關 position which is normally associated with the wood/liver/gall bladder is soggy and weak, it means that the wood *qì* has vacated the original location where it belongs and is now attacking the earth phase.

The same would be true if a wiry quality was found in the left *cùn* 寸 position associated to the heart. It means that liver or gallbladder *qì* is invading the heart, so the mother is violating the child phase. In the case of the wood violating the earth, this is *kè* 剋/control cycle but both of these are not normative. So in *Nán Jīng* 難經 2, the *yīn* in the *yáng* position of the *cùn* 寸 or *yáng* in the *chǐ* 尺 foot position in the *yīn* is considered to be an abnormal juxtaposition or *jué* 厥/inversion. Now in Difficult Issue 20 of the *Nán Jīng* 難經, we find *yáng* qualities of the vessels in the *yīn* section in the interior, that means *yáng* is seizing the *yīn* not in its proper place and in a sense *yīn* and *yáng* have been turned upside down. If there is a rough, short vessel quality, the *yīn qì* 陰氣 is now appearing at the *yáng* level at the top, so it's mixing in the opposite way. This is similar to the earlier example of wood *qì* seizing earth. If *yáng qì* 陽氣 doubles it is very replete and very strong, creating a double *yáng* condition, resulting in a condition we call *kuáng* 狂 or madness. If the *yīn qì* 陰氣 doubles the resulting conditions it is what Unschuld translates "peak illness," *diān* 癲/withdrawal. When the *yáng qì* 陽氣 are lost, or when they are out of control one sees demons. The person becomes a victim of delusion. According to Zhāng Jǐng-yuè 張景岳, "If *shén* 神 and *zhì* 志 are unbalanced, the pathogens establish themselves in turn, then ghosts/*guǐ* 鬼 are generated in the heart."[1] Based on the insights of Zhāng Jǐng-yuè's 張景岳 description, my understanding of *guǐ* 鬼 here means delusional thoughts that obscure clear thinking and emotions. When the *yīn qì* 陰氣 is lost, one's eyes lose the ability to have vision. We often will see this in those today with what we call in general bipolar disorder. Where a person goes through a very *yáng* stage and is very hot, sweaty, agitated, with red eyes and tongue and have a

---

1   Rossi 2007: 272

vessel quality that is flooding *yáng* pulse, and will eventually exhaust their *yáng qì* 陽氣 and the condition will transform into a *yīn* state. The vessel movement is deep, the patient withdraws, and it is as if their eyes withdraw back into their head and they become mute.

CHAPTER 16

NÁN JĪNG 難經 22 AND THE MÀI JĪNG'S 脈經 SHÍ GUÀI MÀI 十怪脈/TEN STRANGE VESSEL MOVEMENTS

Distinguishing Disease of Qì and Blood in Vessel Discrimination and Keys to Diagnosing Serious Disorders

Here we are talking about the concept of *shì dòng* 是動, being stirred up or excited. This Difficult Issue differentiates between diseases of *qì* and blood and how they are influenced by *biǎo xié* 表邪/exterior evils. This is related to *wèi qì* 衛氣/defense *qì* and *yíng qì* 營氣/construction *qì*, which includes blood and the fluids. When you see the term *dòng* 動/stirring or to excite, it means that the *qì* is the first aspect that is affected by any external influence, including wind, cold, damp, warmth, fire, or dryness. If the exterior is vacuous, the exterior evil may penetrate directly into the interior which is what the *Shāng Hán Lùn* 傷寒論 calls a direct strike/*zhí zhòng* 直中. As the *wèi qì* 衛氣/defense *qì* attempts to eliminate the evil, it must activate the *yáng* channels. When activated, defense *qì* will make the vessel dynamic more rapid and floating. If the illness is not rectified at the level of the *yáng qì*, it will influence the *yīn* sector, including the fluids and xuè 血/blood. So, in summary, the qì is affected initially and if it is not resolved it will go to the yīn layer.

In the Shāng Hán Lùn 傷寒論, it states that xié qì 邪氣/evil qì enters the yīn stages and the internal viscera, blood, and fluids. The problem is when it enters the blood and fluids, this is now categorized as an internal disease and it becomes much more difficult to expel this disease to the exterior. Only the yáng channels have exit routes to the exterior, and in the yáng channel stages, where we use the methods of sweating/hàn fǎ 汗法, precipitation/xià fǎ 下法, purging, vomiting/tù fǎ 吐法, and disinhibiting urination/lì xiǎo biàn 利小便 to expel the xié qì 邪氣/evil qì. When illness is in the yīn stages, one externalizes the xié qì 邪氣/evil qì by strengthening the internal viscera, applying hé fǎ 和法/harmonization to bring the evils to the surface again. The Shāng Hán Lùn 傷寒論 goes on to explain that these conditions occur when the qì is stagnant, in other words when the qì of the body is not flowing correctly. I would add that when the qì is vacuous, when there is insufficient wèi qì 衛氣 to defend the body or if there is stasis of the blood (if the blood and the fluids are not flowing or moving yíng qì 營氣), this also allows evils to lodge in it as well. This is one of the general strategies of Chinese medicine, to regulate and move qì and blood. Lǐ Shí-zhēn 李時珍 explains that within the qì kǒu 氣口/wrist opening, the "yīn and yáng intersect, and it is divided into five positions, front and back, left and right (and the middle), each of which has its master. The upper, lower and middle positions are then divided into the nine pathways. When the vessel is examined in this manner, one may know where the disease pathogen lies."[2]

The Mài Jīng 脈經 is considered to be the major classic on which vessel dynamics is based, compiled by Wáng Shū-hē 王叔和 in the same era that he compiled the Shāng Hán

---

2   Chace, Shima, and Li 2010:161

Lùn 傷寒論. The *Shāng Hán Lùn* 傷寒論, of course, also has a large portion devoted to vessel diagnosis, and the author of the *Nán Jīng* 難經 appears to reference both texts, although it is difficult to determine exactly where and how. The *Mài Jīng* 脈經 establishes the daily cycles of vessel dynamics:

> In terms of the pulse, dawn is referred to as *tài yáng* 太陽, midday as *yáng míng* 陽明, late afternoon as *shào yáng* 少陽, twilight as *shào yīn* 少陰, midnight as *tài yīn* 太陰, and cocks crow as *jué yīn* 厥陰. These are the three *yīn* and three *yáng* in connection with time.[3]

In addition, the *Mài Jīng* 脈經 establishes what a *zhèng* 正/correct vessel dynamic looks like. Before we can understand how illnesses are revealed in vessel dynamics, we first need to understand normal vessel qualities, and how chronobiology based on day/night, lunar, solar, and seasonal cycles influences what we feel. Once we've established these qualities, we then can differentiate the different influences from inside and outside the body/mind:

> In spring, (there) should appear the liver pulse. If, instead, a spleen or lung pulse appears, there is damage. In summer, there should appear the heart pulse. If, instead, a kidney or lung pulse appears, there is damage. In autumn, there should appear the lung pulse. If instead, a liver or heart pulse appears, there is damage. In winter, there should appear the kidney pulse. If instead, a heart or spleen pulse appears, there is damage.[4]

Wáng Shū-Hé 王叔和 further establishes the qualities exhibited in vessel dynamics of severe disturbances to *yīn* and *yáng qì*: "On examination, death pulse *qi* may feel like a flock of birds

---

3 Wang and Yang 2002: 130
4 Wang and Yang 2002: 112

gathering, a tied horse galloping to and fro by a river, or a rock falling from a precipice."[5]

The *Mài Jīng* 脈經 also established a system of reading distal proximal and central vessel palpation in order to access the *qí jīng bā mài* 奇經八脈/extraordinary vessels, further developed by Lǐ Shí-zhēn 李時珍 in the *Qí Jīng Bā Mài Kǎo* 奇經八脈考 (16th century). While we will not cover extraordinary vessel diagnostics in this text, it is interesting to note that the vessels are not just divided in three parts (*cùn guān chǐ* 寸關尺) lengthwise, but also by width, further expanding the architecture of vessel dynamics. Vessel palpation systems in Ayurvedic and Tibetan medicine also read these three aspects of the vessel as well, although not in terms of of the *qí jīng bā mài* 奇經八脈/ which is exclusively discussed in Chinese medicine.

One essential, and profound teaching of the *Mài Jīng* 脈經 that I've chosen to include here, as they appear so often in our patients with chronic, complex autoimmune disorders, are the *shí guài mài* 十怪脈/ten strange vessel movements. They have tremendous clinical importance, appear frequently, and expand our scope of diagnosis and practice. They indicate either serious, potentially life-threatening diseases, or "visceral death." This means that the functions of the specific *zàng* 臟/ *yīn* viscera, *fǔ* 腑/bowel, or extraordinary *fǔ* 腑 is going "off-line," in other words, the functional/visceral system is failing. If other visceral systems are able to compensate and fulfill those missing functions, the patient will survive, but the systems will be biased in a potentially permanent state of disequilibrium. For example, if the gall bladder is surgically removed, the liver, kidney, and spleen will compensate for the loss, but there will be permanent biasing, leading to risks of symptoms such as weight gain, increased phlegm/damp clogging the vessels, fatigue, and decreased efficiency of ministerial fire circulation, even though the channel function of *shào yáng* 少陽 remains intact.

---

5   Wang and Yang 2002: 141

Wáng Shū-Hé's 王叔和 *Shí Guài Mài* 十怪脈 Ten Strange Vessel Movements

1 *Wū lòu mài* 屋漏脈
Leaking Roof Vessel Movement

This typically manifests in the *guān* 關 position, mainly on the right hand, and feels as if there is a hole in the vessel movement from which essence is dripping downwards at irregular intervals. It is seen commonly in later stages of many cancers.

2 *Què zhuó mài* 雀啄脈
Pecking Sparrow Vessel Movement

This feels like a short "blip," a quick entry and exit with minimal length and depth, urgent with irregular rhythm. It means that the person's *qì* is tenuous. Both of these vessel movement qualities indicate damage to the spleen. The vessel feels wooden or inflexible like steel, indicating that the *yīn* viscera have hardened and no long perform their functions correctly. This vessel movement is often seen in kidney disease.

3 *Tán shí mài* 彈石脈
Flicking Stone Vessel Movement

This is sunken and replete, and has a movement like a flicking stone thrown across a lake, skipping, and stirring up the water. It indicates deep kidney pathology.

4 *Jiě suǒ mài* 解索脈
Untwining Rope Vessel Movement

This vessel movement is common in patients with cancer, autoimmune diseases, or taking multiple medications. Wáng Shū-Hé 王叔和 believed that this vessel movement beats in a chaotic manner, and feels like multiple strands intertwined with each other. I read this as a pulse indicative of "humoral disruption," when the blood, fluids, and *jīng* 精/essence no longer blend together correctly. The vessel dynamics are tight in some places, loose in others, and seems to move in an uneven manner.

5 *Xiā yóu mài* 蝦游脈
Darting Shrimp Vessel Movement

Rises slowly and leisurely, but quickly retreats and disappears (flicks), rising again after a period of time. It is fluttery, has irregular shape and rhythm. This points to instability of *jīng* 精/essence. The depleted essence does not fill the channels. It indicates damage to the kidney, bladder or *mìng mén* 命門/life gate. This can be associated with the *jué yīn* 厥陰 stage of illness as described in the *Shāng Hán Lùn* 傷寒論, where *yīn* and *yáng* are separating, leading to loss of communication of the *zàng* 臟/viscera and *fǔ* 腑/bowels, *yíng* 營 and *wèi* 衛, construction and defense.

6 *Yú xiáng mài* 魚翔脈
Fish Wavering Vessel Movement

This vessel movement has a slow and delayed arrival and then quickly disappears. It is fixed in place, with movement only in the head and tail, usually *cùn* 寸 and *chǐ* 尺 positions, while fixed in the *guān* 關 position. This points to deep stasis of blood blocking movement of blood and *qì* between upper, middle, and lower burners.

7 *Má cù mài* 麻促脈
Frenzied Sesame Seed Vessel Movement

Like tiny seeds under the finger, faint and fine, urgent, skipping, and chaotic (usually in all positions). This indicates loss of essence, damage to *shào yīn* 少陰/heart and kidney, seen in late stages of autoimmune disease or cancer, after much bombardment by surgery, drug therapies, or serious heart issues.

8 Yǎn dāo mài 偃刀脈
Upturned Knife Vessel Movement

This feels like a knife with the blade pointing upwards, fine, and very wiry, as if one could get a paper cut from palpating the vessel. This vessel movement is similar to what is described in *Nán Jīng* 難經 15 as a visceral vessel movement for wood/liver, indicating hyperactivity of the viscus, before it expires, something like the flaring up of a candle flame before it dies out. I find this vessel movement common in patients with liver/gall bladder pathologies, especially when there are extreme emotional expressions and situations.

9 Fǔ fèi mài 釜沸脈
Seething Cauldron Vessel Movement

Extremely rapid and floating, all outward movement with no inward movement. The lung *qì* is floating up and outwards, vital *qì* is being lost. This vessel movement will often be seen in lung disorders. I've observed it in lung cancer patients in middle to late stages, when the lungs are unable to grasp the *qì*.

10 Zhuàn dòu mài 轉豆脈
Spinning Bean Vessel Movement

Comes and goes away, elusively like a spinning bean. It feels like a vibrating string and is often felt in patients with neurological disorders such as multiple sclerosis or Parkinson's disease. This vessel movement is most common in the chi positions, indicating damage to the kidney *qì*.

One should always calculate the strange vessel movements by measuring against the *zhèng qì* 正氣/upright *qì* of the patient. This will give the physician knowledge on the severity and depth of the disease.

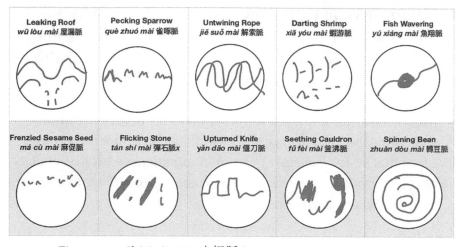

Figure 16.1: Shí Guài Mài 十怪脈/Ten Strange Vessel Movements

CHAPTER 17

NÀN JĪNG 難經 58 AND SHĀNG HÁN LÙN 傷寒論 VESSEL DYNAMICS

There are chapters in the *Nàn Jīng* 難經 that mention vessel dynamics in addition to the first 22 difficulties; for example, *Nàn Jīng* 難經 Difficult Issue 24, which further clarifies *Nàn Jīng* 難經 8, both discussing the severance of the vessels from the kidney *mìng mén* 命門/life gate fire. *Nàn Jīng* 難經 36 discusses the *mìng mén* 命門/life gate, specifically in terms of the vessel positions in the *chǐ* 尺/foot position. In Difficult Issue 58, we find a discussion of *shāng hán* 傷寒/cold damage as it applies to vessel dynamics. In the *Shāng Hán Lùn* 傷寒論, we see that *shāng hán* 傷寒/cold damage has been used as a specific disease pattern associated with *tài yáng bìng* 太陽病/greater *yáng* disease, treated by the *má huáng* 麻黄/*Ephedrae Herba* family of formulas, with floating, tight vessel dynamic, body aches, chills, heat effusion, stuffy nose, and lack of sweating. In *Nàn Jīng* 難經 58, *shāng hán* 傷寒 is categorized as a technical term which includes five types of *wài gǎn* 外感/external contraction. This is similar to the *Shāng Hán Lùn's* 傷寒論 classification of three types of *wài gǎn* 外感 as types of *shāng hán* 傷寒 (including *wēn bìng* 溫病/warm disease and *zhòng fēng* 中風/wind strike). The *Nàn Jīng* 難經 and *Shāng Hán Lùn* 傷寒論 were compiled roughly at the same time and according to Paul Unschuld form similar sources from texts which are no longer available and authors who are no longer named. Of interest is that the five types of cold damage correspond with five phases, which is the central principle along with *yīn yǎng* in the *Nàn Jīng* 難經 text.

The five types of *shāng hán* 傷寒 are as follows:

1. Struck by wind (*zhòng fēng* 中風)

2. Harmed by cold (*shāng hán* 傷寒)

3. Moisture (damp) and warmth (*shī wēn* 濕溫)

4. Heat disease (*rè bìng* 熱病)

5. Warmth disease (*wēn bìng* 溫病).

In each category, there are different signs and symptoms (Figure 17.1 differentiates these). Similarly, the *Shāng Hán Lùn* 傷寒論 discusses the importance of differentiating different stages of illness. For example, a *shāng hán* 傷寒/damage by cold is cured by using a sweating method. However, if the illness is in the large intestine and stomach, i.e. *yáng míng fǔ zhèng* 陽明腑證/ *yáng* brightness bowel pattern, that is when we would use a *dà huáng* 大黃/*Rhei Radix et Rhizoma* formula to *xià* 下/precipitate the bowel. However, if this method which evacuates an internal repletion method is used for an exterior condition, it would weaken the exterior, causing the illness to progress inward at a faster rate than it otherwise would under the circumstances. The *Nàn Jīng* 難經 says that *xià* 下/precipitation would lead to death, although usually this doesn't occur in modern times. In ancient times, it is possible that the treatments were so strong that precipitation was used in extreme conditions, with higher risks entailed. The text goes on to explain how to diagnose each of the tissues that might be affected by these illnesses, such as the skin, body hair, flesh (associated with spleen), lips and tongue, and bones (associated with the kidney). For each of these descriptions of vessel dynamics, we can then choose herbal medicine treatment or acupuncture/moxibustion accordingly.

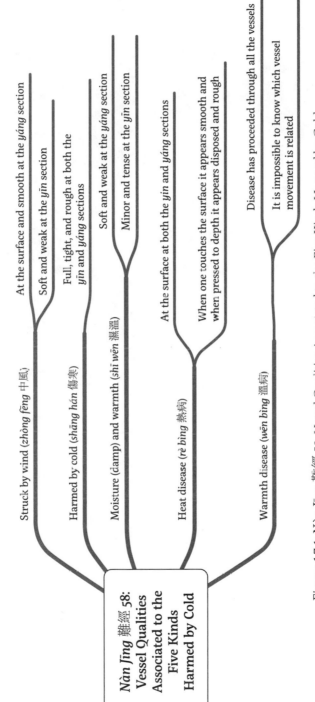

Figure 17.1: Nàn Jīng 難經 58: Vessel Qualities Associated to the Five Kinds Harmed by Cold

CHAPTER 18

VESSEL DYNAMICS AND CASE HISTORIES

Applying Nàn Jīng 難經 Vessel Dynamics to Diagnosis and Treatment

Wǔ xíng xué 五行學/five phase theory was originally developed in the Warring States era (475–221 BCE), by Zou Yǎn 鄒衍, founder of the Naturalist School. As applied in Chinese medicine, I utilize the specific strategies of seeing the *wǔ zàng* 五臟/five *yīn* viscera in terms of familial relationships. Using Confucian logic, where normative behavior brings health, and chaotic, out-of-order behavior brings illness, we can see dysfunctional behavior of visceral systems through the vessel dynamics. In *Nàn Jīng* 難經 49 and 50, the dynamics of internal evils are described as depletion evils, repletion evils, robber evils, weakness evils, and *zhèng xié* 正邪/correct (regular) evils. Each of the five phases can be damaged by their associated damages, (kidneys by humidity, lungs by cold, spleen by irregular eating/drinking and exhaustion, heart by heat, liver by wind), and then be transferred to other phases/viscera by the *shēng* 生/generating or *kè* 剋/control cycle. Each of the phases and viscera have their normative *qì* associated with each season, and reflected in the vessel dynamics, abdominal palpation, and other signs and symptoms. Sometimes, these qualities may appear in other viscera and are reflected in terms of vessel dynamics and symptoms, as in the first case history below, where the normal wiry quality of the liver appears on the right wrist, and the more soggy quality associated with the spleen appears on the left wrist.

Case history 1

A 67-year-old woman, diagnosed with ovarian cancer. The right hand vessel dynamic was very wiry, strong, and rapid. The left hand vessel was very soggy. The patient had chemotherapy the previous week, and tests showed a tumor in the liver along with lymphatic tumors. She suffered diarrhea after (chemotherapy) treatment, as Chinese medical diagnosis revealed that the liver was being "attacked" by the chemotherapy. As the tumor disintegrated, *xié qì* 邪氣/evil *qì* was directed to the spleen/stomach according to five phase theory, explaining the wiry quality on the right hand. Here, the spleen/stomach has absorbed the attacking replete liver *qì*, and taken it downwards to metal (large intestine), leading to strong diarrhea. The liver (wood) also shunted *xié qì* 邪氣/evil *qì* to the heart (replete fire), leading to mouth and tongue sores. The tongue had a dark red tip, body pale. The acupuncture treatment strategy was to balance fire and water in *shào yīn* 少陰. Needling points Kid 2 (*rán gǔ* 然谷) and H 3 (*shào hǎi* 少海) on alternate sides of body, Liv 2 (*xíng jiān* 行間) and Per 3 (*qū zé* 曲澤), alternate sides, St. 36 (*zú sān lǐ* 足三里) with moxa, Liv 13 (*zhāng mén* 章門) (abdomen on palpation very hard and distended), Ren 5 (*shí mén* 石門), moxa on needle, Du 20 (*bǎi huì* 百會). I gave the herbal formula *dāng guī sì nì jiā wú zhū yú shēng jiāng tāng* 當歸四逆加吳茱萸生薑湯/*Chinese Angelica Counterflow Cold Decoction Plus Evodia and Fresh Ginger* to protect the extremities, warm and transform blood, and keep open the circulatory pathways. I also gave *huáng qí rén shēn tāng* 黃耆人參湯/*Astragalus and Ginseng Decoction* to supplement the spleen and stomach, while gently regulating the liver *qì*. The formulas were alternated, the first formula taken in the afternoon and evening, the second in the morning on waking.

Case history 2

A middle-aged male, in the late stages of bronchitis. His hands felt hot and puffy. For two weeks, at the back of his throat he had irritation, post-nasal drip, and a feeling of abdominal stagnation. As it was winter in California, his home was cold inside due to the lack of insulation and inefficient heating in houses in warm climates. On a visit to his family in a desert agricultural region, he had a reaction to pesticide exposure. The next day, he felt a cold with a productive cough, with yellow/green mucous, shallow breath, and a lack of sensation in the abdominal area. His ankles were swollen, and he felt abdominal stagnation from excessive sitting and writing. His vessel diagnosis indicated water and *xuè* 血/blood confining each other in the deep (*yīn*) aspect of the vessels. The left side was stronger, the right side weaker, and the right *cùn* position was large and expanded. His tongue had a dark body with coating at the center and back. His diagnosis was *yáng míng* 陽明 body type, water and fire contending in *shào yīn* 少陰, phlegm-heat congealing in the lungs. His herbal prescription was a combination of *qīng fèi tang* 清肺湯/*Clear the Lungs Decoction* and *xiǎo chái hú tāng* 小柴胡湯/*Minor Bupleurum Decoction*. I needled Lu 5 (*chǐ zé* 尺澤) and Lu 10 (*yú jì* 魚際) on the right, Kid 7 (*fù liū* 復溜) on the left, St. 40 (*fēng lóng* 豐隆) on the right, GB 40 (*qiū xū* 丘墟) on the left, TB 4 (*yáng chí* 陽池) on the right.

Case history 3

A patient diagnosed with celiac disease ten months before coming in. She suffered from anxiety, which had worsened since her mother had just passed away, and was raised in a home with ten brothers and sisters. She retained water, felt "arthritic," with tight joints, aggravated by several years of intensive gym workouts, which she had recently curtailed. Her sleep was disturbed, and there was lots of emotional stress. Her father died three years ago, and she had recently been engaged to be married. She had a torn left hip labrum, with no pain from the original injury that occurred three or four years ago. The medial glute was always tight, and there was occasional back pain. The blood pressure was low, with a low resting pulse rate, and she sweated easily and frequently. There were visible, prominent veins on arms and legs. Her mother had lupus. The patient had a sudden period after these had ceased for 15 months. The tongue had a very red tip, with a deep indentation in the lung area, dark red streaks on the sides (Liv/GB area). She had puffy hands, and dark circles under her eyes. Her vessel diagnosis was on the right hand, a "staircase vessel," in other words, weak in the *yīn* (*chǐ* 尺) section, replete in the *yáng cùn* 寸 section. On the left wrist, the *cùn* 寸 and *guān* 關 positions were very replete, hard, and tense. Her diagnosis was *shào yáng* 少陽/*jué yīn* 厥陰 disorder, counterflow/*nüè qì* 瘧氣, ministerial fire rising to upper burner, water/fire disharmony, wood/earth disharmony. Here, acupuncture treatment was needling alternate sides Kid 2 (*rán gǔ* 然谷) with H 3 (*shào hǎi* 少海) to harmonize *shào yīn* 少陰 water and fire, Sp 4 (*gōng sūn* 公孫) and Per 6 (*nèi guān* 內關) to harmonize *chōng mài* 衝脈, Liv 13 (*zhāng mén* 章門) to harmonize liver and spleen, Ren 5 (*shí mén* 石門) with moxa to warm *dān tián* 丹田 and triple burner fluid dynamics, Du 20 (*bǎi huì* 百會) and hinting to calm the *shén* 神. Her first herbal prescription was *chái hú guì zhī tāng* 柴胡桂枝湯/*Bupleurum and Cinnamon Twig Decoction*.

Case history 4

A patient complaining of low energy, especially after sex, erectile dysfunction, hypertension, a dependence on coffee with several cups in the morning to get going. The patient's tongue was geographic, very irritated, and red with possible sores. The vessel dynamics revealed a hard, "rock-like" core with a damp, muddy periphery. I interpreted this as damage to kidney essence with damp heat brewing in the lower burner. On the left side, a *cùn* 寸 heart spike, with no strength at the depth or support from the *chǐ* 尺/kidney. The *guān* 關 position revealed a disappearing *jué yīn* 厥陰 vessel, with a fragmented gall bladder vessel at the surface. The *chǐ* 尺 position was that the *chǐ* 尺 positions on both sides were weak. I gave the patient a combination of *shèn qì wán* 腎氣丸/*Kidney Qi Pill* and *tiān xióng sǎn* 天雄散/*Tiān Xióng Aconite Powder*[1] in honey pill form, to be taken twice a day with salted water. I added Yaron Seidman's[2] "Fire-Water" formula in liquid extract, containing two types of *ròu guì* 肉桂/*Cinnamomi Cortex, shēng jiāng* 生薑/*Zingiberis Rhizoma Recens, zhì gān cǎo* 炙甘草/*Glycyrrhizae Radix praeparata,* and *ròu dòu kòu* 肉豆蔻/*Myristicae Semen.* One to two droppers per day. I needled on the back Bl 11 (*dà zhù* 大杼), Bl 14 (*jué yīn shù* 厥陰俞), Bl 23 (*shèn shù* 腎俞) with direct moxa, Bl 28 (*páng guāng shù* 膀胱俞), and Kid 10 (*yīn gǔ* 陰谷). On the front, I needled GB 1 (*tóng zǐ liáo* 瞳子髎), TB 4 (*yáng chí* 陽池) on left, GB 40 (*qiū xū* 坵墟) on right, Liv 3 (*tài chōng* 太衝) on left, Per 7 (*dà líng* 大陵) on right, Ren 6 (*qì hǎi* 氣海) with moxa, GB 34 (*yáng líng quán* 陽陵泉), and Liv 8 (*qū quán* 曲泉), the treatment for kidney and liver divergent vessels.

Case history 5

A woman in her early 50s, diagnosed with myasthenia gravis. The patient had had multiple upper cervical spine surgeries to C 3–7, the first one in 1999. The right arm was immobilized, then diagnosed with myasthenia in April 2003. She had an enlarged thymus that was pushing against the blood vessels. She had congenital bone issues, with bones fused together, and had had an experimental stem cell transplant at the University of California in San Diego in 2007, with a lot of chemotherapy beforehand. She had had multiple crises from infections. She had ongoing fatigue, and couldn't exercise without weakening,

---

1   This is a *Jīn Guì Yào Lüè* 金匱要略 found in chapter 6 line 8.
2   For more information about Yaron Seidman and his Fire-Water formula visit his website at www.hunyuanacademy.com

although she looked quite trim and fit. She lived with her mother and stepfather, which she felt was a very uncomfortable arrangement. She had had her uvula, adenoids and tonsils removed as a child, due to a history of chronic strep throats. She was on multiple medications, including hormones, pain medications, and Dilaudid, two to three times a day. Her hands and feet were cold. The fusion at C 6–7 was considered to have "failed." She was given retuxan last year. Her tongue was tender and dark red. Vessel dynamics were on the right slightly rapid, a very weak chǐ 尺 vessel, upper guān 關 (stomach) spike, pushing on diaphragm, crowding the cùn 寸 position. On the left, the cùn 寸/guān 關 vessel were very tight, the chǐ 尺 vessel small deep and contracted. Her treatment was needling GB 1 (tóng zǐ liáo 瞳子髎) bilaterally, Liv 13 (zhāng mén 章門) on the left, Liv 3 (tài chōng 太衝) on left, Per 7 (dà líng 大陵) on right, TB 4 (yáng chí 陽池) on right, GB 40 (qiū xū 坵墟) on left, Ren 5 (shí mén 石門) with moxa, GB 34 (yáng líng quán 陽陵泉) on the right, and Liv 8 (qū quán 曲泉) on the left, Her prescription was dāng guī sì nì jiā wú zhū yú shēng jiāng tāng 當歸四逆加吳茱萸生薑湯/Chinese Angelica Counterflow Cold Decoction Plus Evodia and Fresh Ginger. This case was a long-term treatment situation, and I have only provided the first diagnosis and recorded treatment here.

Case history 6

A 67-year-old woman suffering from high stress, taking care of her elderly and sick mother. She previously has been treated by me for a range of gastrointestinal disorders, including appendicitis, headaches, bloating, fatigue, and other issues. (I originally picked up the appendicitis from a painful, bloated abdomen, rapid slippery vessel dynamic, and greasy tongue coating. I gave her a treatment and then sent her in to be checked for appendicitis, which required surgery.) After her recent stress, she exhibited a remarkable pulse pattern where the left guān 關/gall bladder position was highly wiry, replete, and externally flooding. All other pulses were contracted and inhibited, like small beads. Her tongue exhibited a one-sided coating and red tip, also indicating issues with the gall bladder. I advised the patient on stress management, prescribed *chái hú shū gān tang* 柴胡疏肝湯/*Bupleurum Decoction to Dredge the Liver,* and administered acupuncture treatment, including GB 1 (*tóng zǐ liáo* 瞳子髎), Liv 3 (*tài chōng* 太衝)/Liv 8 (*qū quán* 曲泉)/Per 7 (*dà líng* 大陵), TB 4 (*yáng chí* 陽池)/GB 40 (*qiū xū* 坵墟)/34 (*yáng líng quán* 陽陵泉), Liv 13 (*zhāng mén* 章門), Ren 5 (*shí mén* 石門) with moxa, Du 20 (*bǎi huì* 百會), *yìn táng* 印堂. She felt much relief after treatment, and her vessel dynamics normalized.

Vessel Dynamic Architecture: Understanding the Diagnostic Grid Chart

Sine Wave

All movements in the vessels have amplitude, a high (zenith) point of maximum *yáng*, a deep (nadir) *yīn* valley, wave sets (close/crowded, well spaced, fast and slow), and regular or irregular movements. *Cùn* 寸/*guān* 關/*chǐ* 尺: in measuring the three positions under the three fingers, we read whether the positions are filled or empty, replete above/empty below, crowded or well spaced, *cháng* 長/long or *duǎn* 短/short.

Timing

This includes the relationship of vessel dynamics to breathing rhythms, expressed as speed, relationship to the timing and *yīn*/*yáng* expansion/contraction of the *wǔ zàng* 五臟/five *yīn* visceral systems, speed of *qì* flow in the channels, and how vessel dynamics coincide time-wise with other forms of diagnosis; for example, tongue and abdominal palpation often show slower rates of change than vessel movements.

Mirror/Reflections

Each diagnostic method and its information reflects the others. The *Nán Jīng* 難經 speaks about the *sè* 色/complexion needing to mirror findings in the vessel dynamics. In turn, we listen to the sound and rhythm of the voice, examine handwriting, watch the patient's breathing, and, of most concern, view the *shén* 神/spirit reflected in the eyes. *Sù Wèn* 素問 17 tells us when we palpate vessel dynamics at dawn, to look up at the eyes to see the root condition of the patient.

Vessel Dimensions

This means to examine the volume of blood, fluids, essence, and *qì* in the vessel, their clear or clouded movements, depth/thickness, *yáng*/surface and *yīn*/interior regions, as well as the *sān jiāo* 三膲/three dynamic "burning/metabolic spaces."

Three Bodies

These are described in *Returning to the Source: Han Dynasty Medical Classics in Modern Clinical Practice*. To summarize, the sentimental body has to do with the relationship of the *qíng* 情/emotions with the *zàng* 臟/viscera. The ecological body is the modern traditional Chinese medicine body of internal climates and terrain, areas of dampness, heat, cold, dryness, and wind, whether intrinsic to the body or pathological. The architectural body is the multi-dimensional cube formed by the *jīng luò* 經絡, its foundation being the *qí jīng bā mài* 奇經八脈/eight extraordinary vessels, filled by the 12 regular channels, and bridged by the *bié* 別/divergent and *luò* 絡/network vessels. Just as the body has depth, height, above, below, inside and outside, back and front, so are these qualities reflected in vessel dynamics.

Vessel Dynamic Architecture

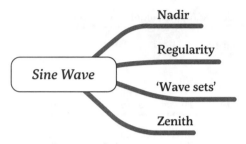

Sine Wave
- Nadir
- Regularity
- 'Wave sets'
- Zenith

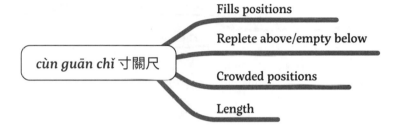

cùn guān chǐ 寸關尺
- Fills positions
- Replete above/empty below
- Crowded positions
- Length

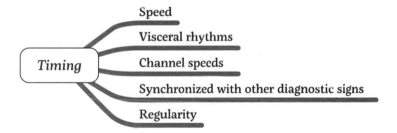

Timing
- Speed
- Visceral rhythms
- Channel speeds
- Synchronized with other diagnostic signs
- Regularity

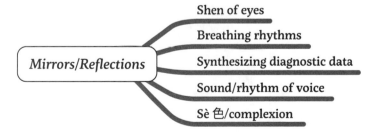

Mirrors/Reflections
- Shen of eyes
- Breathing rhythms
- Synthesizing diagnostic data
- Sound/rhythm of voice
- Sè 色/complexion

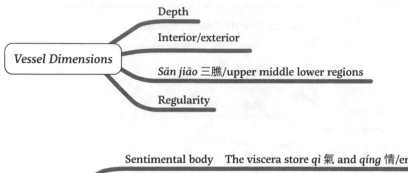

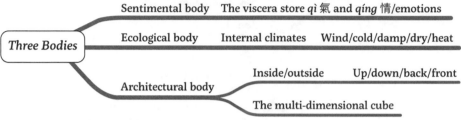

Appendix Figure I.1

28 Traditional Vessel Qualities

Here is a representation of my hand-drawn diagrams for each of the 28 traditional vessel qualities as I've felt them in my daily practice, inspired by diagrams from earlier eras in Chinese medical history.

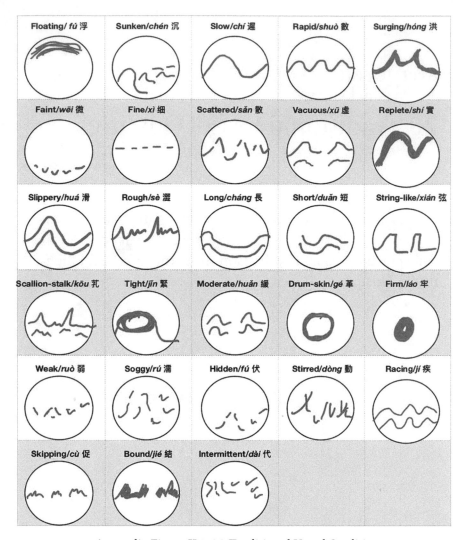

Appendix Figure II.1: 28 Traditional Vessel Qualities

Glossary of Terms

biǎo xié 表邪 *Exterior evils*

bié mài 別脈 *Divergent vessels*

bèi shù xué 背俞穴 *Back-shu points*

biàn 變 *Change*

biàn huà 變化 *Transformation, to change*

bǔ 補 *Supplementation*

cháng 長 *Long quality in the vessel movement*

chén 沉 *Sunken; deep*

cùn kǒu 寸口 *Inch opening; location of the radial pulse*

cùn 寸 *Inch/ guān* 關 *Gate (bar)/ and chǐ* 尺 *Foot (cubit)*

dài 代 *Intermittent*

dòng 動 *Stirring*

fù 覆 *Turnover*

fǔ 腑 *Bowels*

fú mài 浮脈 *Floating pulse*

gé 格 *Barrier*

hàn fǎ 汗法 *Sweating*

hé xué 合穴 *Sea points*

jié mài 結脈 *Bound pulse*

jīn 筋 *Sinews*

jīn jīng 筋經 *Sinew channels*

jīn yè 津液 *Fluids*

jīng 精 *Essence; that which is responsible for growth, development, and reproduction, and determines the strength of the constitution jīng luò* 經絡 *Channels and network (connecting) vessels*

jīng mài 經脈 *Channel/vessel system*

jīng qì 精氣 *Essential qi; any essential element of the body (blood, qi, fluid, essence); specifically, the acquired essence and the essence stored by the viscera and dissociable from the essential qi that is stored by the kidney and used in reproduction*

jǐng xué 井穴/ *Well points*

jué 厥 *Inversion*

kè 剋 *Control; restrain (five phase cycle)*

kè qì 客氣 *Guest qi*

láng gān 琅玕 *Jade-like stone*

láo 牢 *Firm*

lǐ lùn 理論 *Theory/principle*

lì xiǎo biàn 利小便 *Disinhibiting urination*

luò mài 絡脈 *Network vessels*

mài 脈 *Vessels/pulses*

mài xiàng 脈象 *Vessel imagery*

mài zhěn 脈診 *Vessel examination*

mìng mén 命門 *Life gate*

mìng mén huǒ 命門火 *Life gate fire*

nèi shāng 內傷 *Internal damage; internal injury*

nì 逆 *To oppose, go against/counter-flow, flow counter to the normal direction*

qì 氣 *That which animates, transforms and maintains all life; often translated as energy or vital energy. A fundamental concept in Chinese medicine*

qì huà 氣化 *Qi transformation; the movement, mutation, and conversion of qi*

qí jīng bā mài 奇經八脈 *Eight extraordinary vessels*

qīng qì 氣 *Clear qi*

rè bìng 熱病 *Heat disease*

rén qì 人氣 *Humanity; man qi*

rén yíng 人迎 *Man's prognosis; the pulsating vessel at the sides of the neck*

ròu 肉 *Flesh*

ruò 弱 *Soft but replete quality*

sǎn 散 *Scattered pulse, dissipated pulse*

sān bù 三部 *Three sectors*

sān jiāo 三焦 *Three burners/three heaters; one of the six fu*

sān yáng 三陽 *Three yáng*

sān yīn 三陰 *Three yīn*

sè 色 *Complexion color*

sè 澀 *Choppy, rough*

shāng 傷 *Damaged*

shāng hán 傷寒 *Cold damage*

shén 神 *Spirit; consciousness*

shēng 生 *Generating cycle*

shí 實 *Repletion*

shì dòng 是動

shí guài mài 十怪脈 *Ten Strange Vessel Movements*

shí qì 時氣 *Seasonal qì*

shī wēn 濕溫 *Moisture (damp) and warmth*

shí xié 實邪 *Repletion evil*

sǔn 損 *Injury*

tán 痰 *Phlegm*

tù fǎ 吐法 *Vomiting*

wài gǎn 外感 *External contractions*

wáng qì 王氣 *Ruling qì*

wèi qì 衛氣 *Defense qi; the superficially protective aspect of the circulation of qi, that is within the channels defends the body from outside invasion*

wēi xié 微邪 *Weakness evil*

wēn bìng 溫病 *Warm disease*

wǔ shū xué 五输穴 *Five transport points*

wǔ xíng 五行 *The five phases (Wood, Fire, Earth, Metal, Water)*

wǔ xíng biàn zhèng 五行辨證 *Five phase pattern differentiation*

wǔ xíng xué shuō 五行學說 *Five phase theory*

wǔ yùn liù qì 五運六氣 *Five periods and six qi; chronobiology theory*

wǔ zàng 五臟 *Five viscera (heart/xīn 心, liver/gān 肝, spleen/pí 脾, lungs/fèi 肺 and kidneys/shè 腎)*

wǔ zhì 五志 *Five sentiments (emotions)*

xià fǎ 下法 *Precipitation*

xiàng huǒ 相火 *Ministerial fire*

xiè 瀉 *Draining*

xié qì 邪氣 *Evil qi; unhealthy influences that cause disease; pathogenic invasive agent which usually enters the body from the outside*

xū 虛 *Depletion/vacuity*

xū xié 虛邪 *Vacuity evil*

xuè 血 *Blood*

xīn bāo 心包 *Heart envelope master*

xué 穴 *Hole, acupuncture point*

yì 益 *Overflow*

yīn yáng 陰陽 *The two fundamental aspects of the universe; the shady and sunny side of the mountain*

yíng qì 營氣 *Construction, provisioning*

yuán qì 原氣 *Source qi; The basic form of qi in the body, which is made up of a combination of three other forms of qi: the essential qi of the kidney; qi of grain and water; derived through the transformative function of the spleen; and air (great qi) drawn in through the lung*

yuán xué 原穴 *Source hole*

zàng 臟 *Viscera; viscus, any of the five viscera (lung, kidney, liver, heart, and spleen)*

zàng qì 臟氣 *Visceral qi*

zàng xiàng 臟象 *Visceral manifestation*

zhēn zàng mài 真臟脈 *Genuine visceral movement in the vessels*

zhèng qì 正氣 *Right qi; correct qi; true qi; upright qi*

zhèng xié 正邪 *Correct evil*

zhōng 中 *Center (position associated with dì* 地/ *earth); central, middle*

zhòng fēng 中風 *Wind strike*

zhuó qì 濁氣 *Turbid qi*

zhì 至 *Arrival*

zhì 滯 *Knotted (stagnant)*

zhí zhòng 直中 *Direct strike*

zhǔ qì 主氣 *Host qi; governing qi*

References

Bray, F., Dorofeeva-Lichtmann, V., and Métailié, G. (2007). *Graphics and Text in the Production of Technical Knowledge in China: The Warp and the Weft*. Leiden: Brill.

Chace, C., Shima, M., and Li, S. (2010). *An Exposition on the Eight Extraordinary Vessels: Acupuncture, Alchemy, and Herbal Medicine*. Seattle, WA: Eastland Press.

Dhonden, Y. and Hopkins, J. (1986). *Health through Balance: An Introduction to Tibetan Medicine*. Ithaca, NY: Snow Lion.

Foucault, M. (2003). *The Birth of the Clinic: An Archaeology of Medical Perception* (trans. A. Sheridan). London: Routledge.

Holt, J. (2018). *When Einstein walked with Gödel: Excursions to the Edge of Thought*. New York, NY: Farrar, Straus & Giroux.

Kuriyama, S. (2011). *The Expressiveness of the Body and the Divergence of Greek and Chinese Medicine*. New York, NY: Zone Books.

Legge, J. (n.d.). *Inner Chapters: Nourishing the Lord of Life*. Retrieved from https://ctext.org/zhuangzi/nourishing-the-lord-of-life

Manaka, Y., Itaya, K., and Birch, S. (1995). *Chasing the Dragon's Tail: The Theory and Practice of Acupuncture in the Work of Yoshio Manaka*. Brookline, MA: Paradigm Publications.

Rosenberg, Z. (2018). *Returning to the Source: Han Dynasty Medical Classics in Clinical Practice*. London: Singing Dragon.

Rossi, E. (2007). *Shen: Psycho-emotional Aspects of Chinese Medicine*. Edinburgh: Churchill Livingstone Elsevier.

Solos, I. (2012). *Gold Mirrors and Tongue Reflections: The Cornerstone Classics of Chinese Medicine Tongue Diagnosis*. London: Singing Dragon.

Unschuld, P. (2003, November 11). *The Yellow Emperor's Classics: The Messages of the Huang Di Nei Jing Su Wen and the Nan Jing*. Lecture presented at Pacific Symposium 2003 in San Diego, California.

Unschuld, P. (2016). *Huang Di Nei Jing Ling Shu: The Ancient Classic on Needle Therapy: The Complete Chinese Text with an Annotated English Translation.* Oakland, CA: University of California Press.

Unschuld, P. (2016). *Nan Jing: The Classic of Difficult Issues.* Berkeley, CA: University of California Press.

Unschuld, P. and Tessenow, H. (2011). *Huang Di Nei Jing Su Wen: An Annotated Translation of Huang Di's Inner Classic—Basic Questions, 2 Volumes.* Berkeley, CA: University of California Press.

Wang, S. and Yang, S. (2002). *The Pulse Classic: A Translation of the Mai Jing.* Boulder, CO: Blue Poppy Press.

Wilms, S. (2018). *Humming with Elephants: The Great Treatise on the Resonant Manifestations of Yin and Yang: A Translation and Discussion of Chapter Five of the Yellow Emperor's Inner Classic Plain Questions.* Whidbey Island, WA: Happy Goat Productions.

Wiseman, N. and Ye, F. (1998). *Practical Dictionary of Chinese Medicine.* Taos, NM: Paradigm Press.

Zhuangzi and Watson, B. (1964). *Chuang Tzu. Basic Writings.* New York, NY: Columbia University Press.

Index